BEYOND NEUROPATHY: RECLAIM YOUR LIFE WITH THE WARRIOR PROTOCOL

Dr. Bill Jensen DC
Beyond Neuropathy: Reclaim Your Life with the WARRIOR
Protocol

Published by Spines
ISBN: 979-8-89569-977-5

BEYOND NEUROPATHY: RECLAIM YOUR LIFE WITH THE WARRIOR PROTOCOL

DR. BILL JENSEN DC

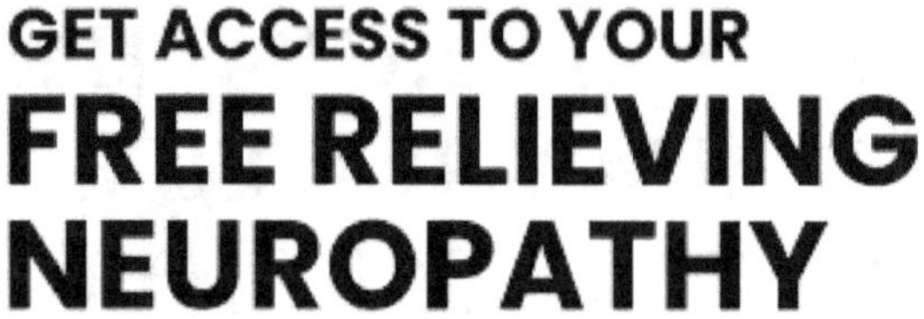

GET ACCESS TO YOUR
FREE RELIEVING
NEUROPATHY
GIFTS BELOW

premier
Wellness Centers

- Neuropathy Health Journal
- Relieving Neuropathy Guide
- 25 Anti-Inflammatory Recipes
- Nerve Damage Quiz
- Free Health Masterclass
- 30-Day Nutrition Plan
- Neuropathy Relief
  Handbook

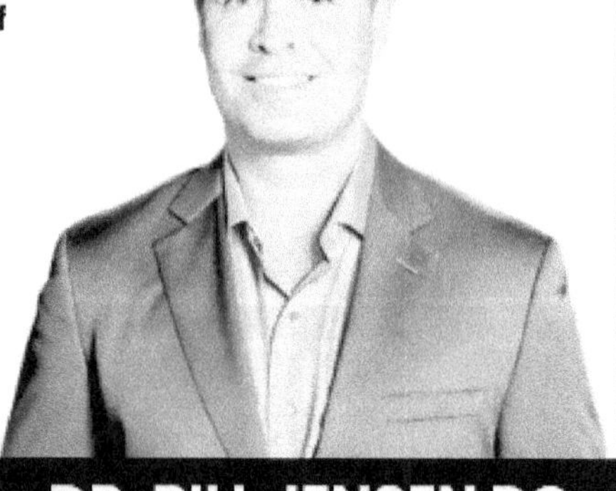

SCAN ME   DR. BILL JENSEN DC

CONTENTS

FOREWORD

When Dr. Bill Jensen, D.C., invited me to pen the foreword for Beyond Neuropathy: Reclaim Your Life with the WARRIOR Protocol, I was deeply honored. Bill and I have crossed paths numerous times through our shared membership in the Driven Docs community, and I've always admired his dedication to providing top-tier care and his unwavering commitment to patient outcomes. However, it was his exploration into the realm of neuropathy that truly captivated me.

As a chiropractor who has worked extensively with individuals with neuropathy, I've seen the profound impact this condition can have on people's lives and their families. The relentless pain, numbness, tingling, and weakness can erode a person's quality of life, leaving them feeling hopeless and isolated. Tragically, many patients are resigned to the belief that neuropathy is a life sentence, a burden they must bear with little hope of relief.

Dr. Jensen, founder and chiropractor at Premier Wellness Centers, refused to accept this narrative for his patients. Through meticulous research, keen clinical observation, and collaboration with his exceptional team at the chiropractic clinic, he pioneered the W.A.R.R.I.O.R. Protocol – a comprehensive and dynamic approach to managing and relieving neuropathy. This protocol isn't just a theoretical framework; it's a proven system that has empowered countless patients to reclaim their lives from the grips of this debilitating condition.

Within these pages, Dr. Jensen will walk you through the intricacies of the WARRIOR Protocol, revealing the insights, techniques, and resources that have made it so remarkably effective. You'll delve into the root causes of neuropathy, discover the significance of individualized treatment plans, and understand the pivotal role lifestyle adjustments play in achieving sustainable results.

This book is more than just a guide to neuropathy management; it's a testament to the transformative power of perseverance, innovation, and an unwavering commitment to patient well-being. Dr. Jensen and his team at PWC are not simply healthcare providers; they are beacons of hope for those grappling with the challenges of neuropathy.

Whether you are a patient navigating the complexities of neuropathy or a healthcare professional seeking to enhance your treatment toolkit, *Beyond Neuropathy* is essential reading. It will challenge your preconceived notions, ignite your passion for healing, and equip you to make a profound impact on the lives of those you serve.

Dr. Cory Frogley, D.C.
Co-Founder, The Data Driven Practice

DISCLAIMER

The information provided in this book is intended for educational purposes only and is not a substitute for professional medical advice. The author and publisher are not liable for any adverse effects or consequences resulting from the use of the information presented herein. Always consult your physician or a qualified healthcare provider regarding any health concerns or before making any decisions related to your health or treatment.

The patient or any other person responsible for payment has the right to refuse to pay, cancel payment, or request a refund for any service, examination, or treatment performed as a result of and within 72 hours of responding to this advertisement for free, discounted, or reduced-fee services. All services, including any offered X-rays or exams, will only be provided if deemed medically necessary. Dr. William Jensen, Doctor of Chiropractic (D.C.), licensed in the state of Florida.

ABOUT THE AUTHOR

My journey to becoming a doctor wasn't a typical one. It began on a wrestling mat when I was just nine years old. A sudden neck injury left me temporarily paralyzed, and the fear I felt in that moment has stayed with me ever since. While I thankfully recovered, the experience sparked a deep fascination with the body's incredible ability to heal.

It was chiropractic care and physical therapy that ultimately put me on the road to recovery, easing the migraines, neck pain, and aching muscles that followed my accident. It was then that I knew I wanted to dedicate my life to helping others find the same relief and regain control of their health.

That passion led me to earn my Doctor of Chiropractic degree and eventually found Premier Wellness Centers. My mission? To make world-class wellness accessible to everyone. I believe that everyone deserves access to the transformative power of chiropractic care, massage, and physical therapy, regardless of their background or financial situation.

Through this book, I'm sharing what I've learned over decades of practice and research, culminating in the development of the W.A.R.R.I.O.R. Protocol. It's my hope that this information empowers you to take control of your neuropathy, find lasting relief, and live your life to the fullest.

Thank you for inviting me on your journey to healing. I'm honored to be a part of it.

Dr. William 'Bill' Jensen, D.C.

LIVING WITH INVISIBLE PAIN: A LOOK INSIDE THE NEUROPATHY EPIDEMIC

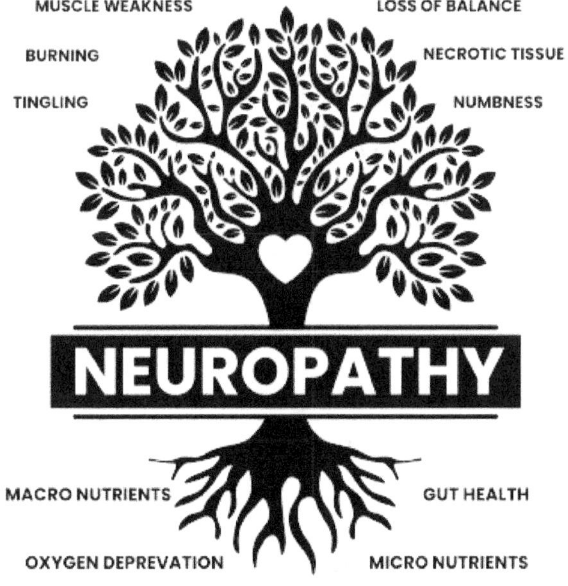

Sarah walked into my office with a hesitant smile, her gaze fixed on the floor. For months, she'd been grappling with the relentless tingling and numbness in her feet, a sensation that had slowly crept up her legs, stealing her stability and making even short walks a challenge. Peripheral neuropathy had become a thief in the night, robbing her of her independence and casting a shadow of fear over her future.

She'd tried everything—medications, acupuncture, even surgery—but nothing seemed to provide lasting relief. The tingling persisted, the numbness spread, and the fear grew. Walking into Premier Wellness Centers, her chiropractic option of choice, her hope was fragile, worn thin by months of disappointment.

But Sarah was determined to reclaim her life. She embraced the WARRIOR Protocol with unwavering commitment, attending her therapy sessions diligently, making dietary changes, and incorporating the stress-reducing techniques we discussed. Week after week, I witnessed a transformation unfold. The hesitant smile became brighter, her gaze lifted, and a glimmer of hope returned to her eyes.

The tingling gradually subsided, the numbness receded, and the strength returned to her legs. She started taking longer walks, rediscovering the joy of simple pleasures she'd once taken for granted. One day, she walked into my office with a radiant smile, tears welling up in her eyes. "Dr. Jensen," she said, "I can feel my feet again! I can walk without fear! I have my life back!"

Witnessing Sarah's transformation is a testament to the power of the WARRIOR Protocol and the resilience of the human body. While every patient's journey is unique, and we can't guarantee similar results for others, Sarah's story exemplifies the profound impact a holistic approach can have on those struggling with neuropathy.

It's a condition that affects millions, often starting with that all-too-familiar "pins and needles" sensation...

Ever had that "pins and needles" sensation after your foot has fallen asleep? Now imagine that feeling sticking around, day in and day out. That's what it's like for millions living with neuropathy. While the sensation itself might start subtly as a mere tingle, it can escalate to a debilitating ache, numbness, and even complete loss of sensation. It's a frustrating condition, often shrouded in mystery and a source of ongoing worry for many.

Imagine a beautiful, flourishing tree. What you see above ground is only part of the story. Deep below, a web of roots provides nourishment and stability. In neuropathy, it's the "roots"—the nerves themselves—that are suffering, malfunctioning, and sending confusing and distorted signals throughout the body. These miscommunications can manifest in tingling sensations, numbness, and pain.

The key to managing neuropathy is understanding that it's often a symptom of a larger issue, just like the wilting leaves of a tree signal problems with its roots. Addressing just the symptoms is not enough; we need to discover and address the underlying cause—be it uncontrolled blood sugar, inflammation, or another factor—to truly find relief. That's the focus of the WARRIOR Protocol—a comprehensive approach to unraveling the mysteries of neuropathy and working towards lasting solutions.

The Root of the Problem: Uncovering the Causes of Neuropathy

Just as a single spark can ignite a forest fire, neuropathy can stem from a variety of sources. While we often associate it with diabetes, it's crucial to remember that this condition is multi-faceted, often developing from a complex interplay of factors. Let's shed some light on some of the most common culprits behind this debilitating condition:

- **Diabetes:** High blood sugar, a hallmark of diabetes, can damage the delicate blood vessels that nourish your nerves. This often leads to a type of neuropathy called diabetic neuropathy, which is particularly prevalent in those struggling to manage their blood sugar levels.

- **Alcoholism:** Excessive alcohol consumption over time can wreak havoc on your body, including your nerves. Alcohol is toxic to nerve tissue and can disrupt nutrient absorption, both of which contribute to alcoholic neuropathy.

- **Vitamin B12 Deficiency:** Think of vitamin B12 as a vital nutrient for healthy nerve function. When your body lacks sufficient B12, it can lead to a specific type of neuropathy called vitamin B12 deficiency neuropathy.

- **Autoimmune Diseases:** In some cases, your own immune system – designed to protect you – can mistakenly attack your nerves as if they were foreign invaders. This can be seen in autoimmune diseases like Guillain-Barré Syndrome, Chronic Inflammatory Demyelinating Polyneuropathy (CIDP), Sjögren's Syndrome, and Lupus.

- **Infections:** Certain infections can trigger an inflammatory response that damages nerves, leading to neuropathy. These infections include Lyme disease, Shingles, and HIV/AIDS.
- **Medications:** While often necessary, certain medications can have unintended side effects, including nerve damage. Chemotherapy drugs, some antibiotics, anticonvulsants, and even certain pain medications can contribute to neuropathy.
- **Physical Injuries:** Trauma to nerves, whether from a car accident, a fall, sports injuries, or even surgery, can disrupt nerve function and lead to neuropathy.
- **Idiopathic Neuropathy:** In some cases, despite extensive testing, the exact cause of neuropathy remains a mystery. This is referred to as idiopathic neuropathy.

As you can see, the path to neuropathy is rarely straightforward. It often involves a combination of risk factors, genetic predisposition, and lifestyle choices. That's why it's crucial to work with a healthcare professional to identify the root cause of *your* neuropathy, allowing for a tailored treatment plan that addresses your unique needs.

Silent Signals: Recognizing the Red Flags of Neuropathy

Neuropathy is a master of disguise, often lurking in the shadows before making its presence known. Its symptoms can be subtle at first, easily mistaken for something else or dismissed as a passing nuisance. But as the condition progresses, those whispers of discomfort can escalate into a chorus of pain, numbness, and dysfunction.

The most commonly recognized symptoms of neuropathy are:

- **Numbness and tingling:** That classic "pins-and-needles" sensation, often felt in the hands and feet, is a telltale sign that your nerves aren't communicating as they should.
- **Pain:** Neuropathy pain can manifest in a variety of ways - from a sharp, shooting pain to a dull, aching throb. Some describe it as a burning sensation, while others experience it as electric shocks or stabbing pains.
- **Weakness:** As nerve damage progresses, you may notice muscle weakness, making it difficult to perform everyday tasks like buttoning your shirt, gripping objects, or climbing stairs.

- **Loss of Coordination and Balance:** Neuropathy can affect your sense of proprioception – your body's ability to know where it is in space. This can lead to clumsiness, difficulty with balance, and an increased risk of falls.

However, neuropathy's reach extends beyond these common symptoms. It can also disrupt the autonomic nervous system, which controls vital functions like heart rate, digestion, and bladder control. This can lead to a range of less commonly recognized symptoms, such as:

- **Changes in heart rate and blood pressure:** You might notice your heart racing or pounding, or you may experience dizziness or lightheadedness due to fluctuating blood pressure.
- **Digestive Issues:** Neuropathy can affect the muscles and nerves that control digestion, leading to nausea, vomiting, constipation, diarrhea, or even difficulty swallowing.
- **Urinary and Bowel Difficulties:** You might find it harder to control your bladder, leading to frequent urination, urgency, or

incontinence. Constipation or bowel incontinence can also occur.

- **Sweating Changes:** Some individuals with neuropathy experience excessive sweating, even when at rest, while others might find themselves sweating less than usual.
- **Sexual Dysfunction:** Neuropathy can interfere with sexual function in both men and women, leading to difficulties with arousal, lubrication, or achieving orgasm.

In severe cases, neuropathy can progress to paralysis and a complete loss of sensation.

Remember, these symptoms can vary widely from person to person and can depend on the type and severity of neuropathy. It's vital to pay attention to your body and report any unusual sensations or changes to your healthcare provider. Early detection and diagnosis are crucial for effective management and improving your long-term outlook.

Riding the Waves: Strategies for Coping with Neuropathy

Living with neuropathy can feel like navigating a stormy sea. Some days are calm, while others bring unexpected waves of pain, fatigue, and frustration. While finding lasting relief often requires addressing the root cause of your neuropathy, there are many effective strategies you can incorporate into your daily life to help you weather the storms and regain control of your well-being.

Embracing a Holistic Approach

True healing goes beyond addressing physical symptoms; it encompasses your emotional and mental well-being too. By adopting a holistic approach, you acknowledge the interconnectedness of your mind, body, and spirit, empowering you to navigate the challenges of neuropathy with greater resilience.

Physical Strategies

- **Exercise:** While it might seem counterintuitive, gentle exercise can be incredibly beneficial for neuropathy. It helps improve blood flow, strengthens muscles, and enhances nerve function. Consult with your doctor or a physical therapist to develop a safe and effective exercise plan tailored to your needs.
- **Rest:** Just as important as exercise is giving your body adequate rest. Fatigue can exacerbate neuropathy symptoms, so

prioritize restful sleep, practice relaxation techniques, and listen to your body when it needs a break.

- **Nutrition:** What you eat has a direct impact on your nerve health. Focus on a nutrient-rich diet, emphasizing whole foods, fruits, vegetables, and lean proteins. Limit processed foods, sugary drinks, and unhealthy fats, as these can contribute to inflammation and worsen symptoms.
- **Alternative Therapies:** Many find relief from neuropathy symptoms through complementary therapies like acupuncture, massage therapy, and chiropractic care. These modalities can help reduce pain, improve circulation, and promote relaxation.

Emotional and Mental Strategies

- **Support Groups:** Connecting with others who understand your journey can be incredibly empowering. Support groups provide a safe space to share your experiences, learn coping mechanisms, and find strength in community.
- **Mindfulness and Meditation:** Practicing mindfulness techniques, such as deep

breathing exercises and meditation, can help you manage pain, reduce stress, and cultivate a greater sense of peace amidst the challenges of neuropathy.

- **Cognitive Behavioral Therapy (CBT):** CBT is a type of therapy that focuses on identifying and changing negative thought patterns and behaviors that can worsen pain perception. It empowers you to develop coping strategies and regain a sense of control over your experience.

- **Gratitude:** Even in the midst of challenges, focusing on gratitude for the good things in your life can shift your perspective and boost your overall well-being. Try keeping a gratitude journal or simply taking a few moments each day to appreciate the simple joys.

Managing neuropathy is a journey, not a race. Be patient with yourself, celebrate small victories, and remember that you are not alone. By embracing a holistic approach and incorporating these coping strategies, you can navigate the waves of neuropathy with greater strength, resilience, and hope.

A New Path Forward: Introducing the WARRIOR Protocol

Neuropathy treatment has traditionally centered around symptom management, often offering temporary relief without addressing the underlying causes. However, the WARRIOR Protocol presents a paradigm shift, focusing on comprehensive care.

This multifaceted approach emphasizes six key pillars, each scientifically grounded and aimed at empowering the body's intrinsic healing mechanisms. Through this innovative strategy, the WARRIOR Protocol seeks to relieve neuropathy and reclaim your overall well-being.

We will now explore each pillar in depth, delving into the supporting research and its adaptability to individual needs. Prepare to embark on a journey towards lasting health and renewed vitality, empowered by the knowledge of the WARRIOR Protocol.

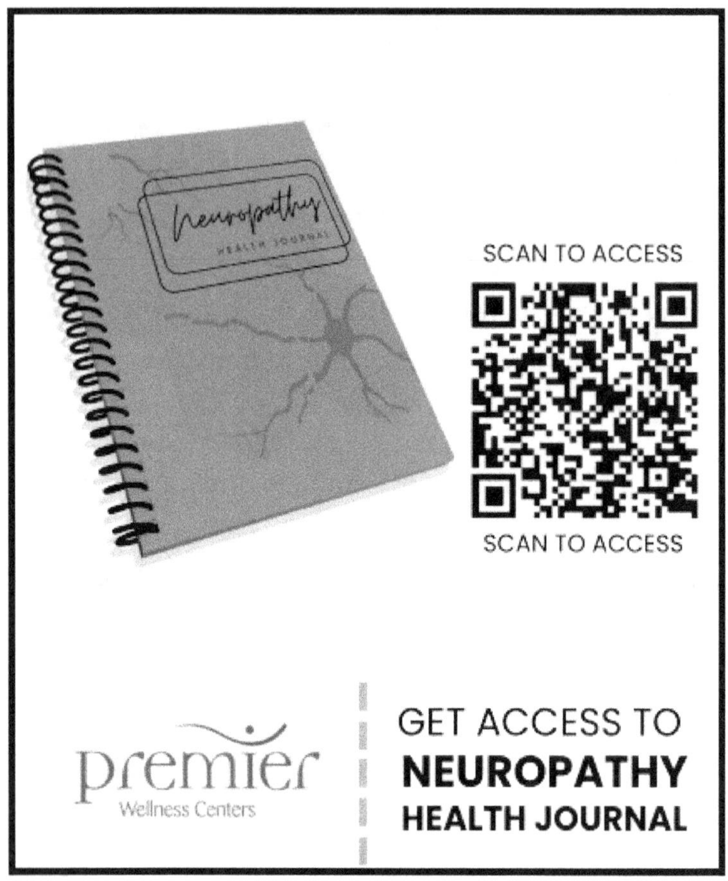

Unlock Your Path to Neuropathy Relief Now: Dial (772) 279-4145 to Speak With a Skilled Neuropathy Professional Today!

Individual results may vary. Please review the disclaimer after the Table of Contents.

2

———

W.A.R.R.I.O.R: A NEW HOPE FOR NEUROPATHY

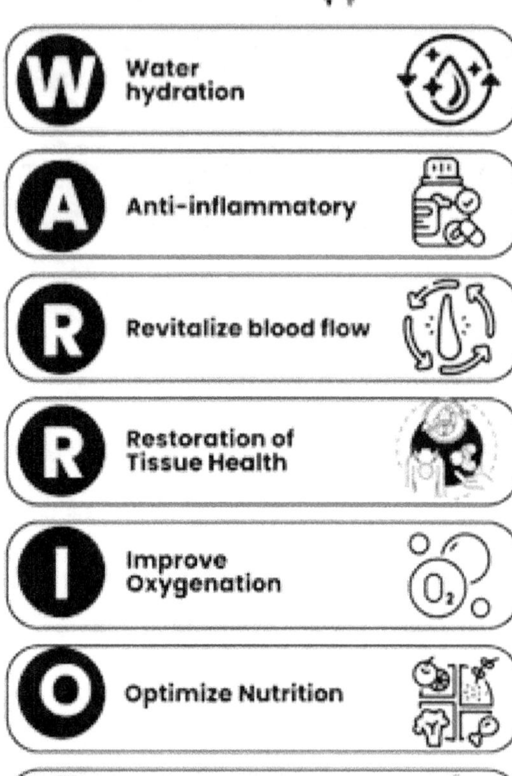
WARRIOR
W Water hydration
A Anti-inflammatory
R Revitalize blood flow
R Restoration of Tissue Health
I Improve Oxygenation
O Optimize Nutrition
R Rehabilitation & Functional Movement

Beyond Band-Aids: Addressing the Shortcomings of Traditional Approaches

If you've sought help for neuropathy, you've likely encountered the limitations of traditional treatment methods. Many of these approaches, while well-intentioned, often fall short of providing lasting relief because they focus on masking the symptoms rather than addressing the root causes. It's like trying to fix a leaky faucet by constantly mopping up the floor—it might provide temporary relief, but it doesn't solve the underlying problem.

Here are some common limitations of conventional neuropathy treatments:

- **Symptom Management Over Root Cause Resolution:** Many traditional approaches rely heavily on medications that primarily mask pain signals without addressing the underlying nerve damage. While pain relief is important, it shouldn't come at the expense of ignoring the source of the problem.
- **Medication Risks and Side Effects:** Medications prescribed for neuropathy often come with a long list of potential side effects, some of which can be as debilitating as the neuropathy itself. Drowsiness, dizziness,

cognitive impairment, and even an increased risk of falls are just a few examples.

- **The One-Size-Fits-All Approach:** Neuropathy is not a one-size-fits-all condition. It manifests differently in each individual, often stemming from a unique combination of factors. Yet, traditional treatments often take a standardized approach, failing to consider the individual's specific needs and health history.

- **Lack of Lifestyle Focus:** While medications might provide temporary relief, lasting solutions often require a more comprehensive approach that includes lifestyle modifications. Sadly, traditional treatments often overlook the importance of nutrition, exercise, stress management, and other lifestyle factors that play a crucial role in nerve health.

This over-reliance on medications and the lack of focus on personalized, holistic care often leave neuropathy sufferers feeling frustrated, unheard, and trapped in a cycle of pain and dependence. This is where the WARRIOR Protocol offers a refreshing and empowering alternative. Instead of simply masking your symptoms, it empowers you to take control of your health and address the root causes of your neuropathy.

Why Symptoms Often Overshadow Solutions

You might be wondering, "If these traditional approaches have limitations, why are they still so prevalent?" It's a complex issue with a multifaceted answer. Several factors contribute to the healthcare system's tendency to focus on symptom management rather than root cause resolution when it comes to neuropathy.

- **The Reductionist Approach:** Modern medicine often operates within a reductionist model, breaking down the body into separate systems and treating symptoms as isolated problems. This approach often fails to recognize the interconnectedness of the body and the complex interplay of factors that contribute to neuropathy.
- **The Complexity of Neuropathy:** As we've discussed, neuropathy can stem from a wide range of causes, making it challenging to pinpoint the root of the problem and develop a targeted treatment plan. This complexity can lead some healthcare providers to resort

to symptom management as a seemingly simpler approach.

- **Time Constraints in Healthcare:** Doctors often face immense time constraints in their practice, leaving limited opportunities for in-depth discussions about lifestyle changes, alternative therapies, and the root causes of chronic conditions like neuropathy.

- **Profit-Driven Healthcare System:** Sadly, the financial incentives within the healthcare system often prioritize expensive medications and procedures over more time-intensive, holistic approaches that emphasize lifestyle modifications and preventative care.

- **Lack of Patient Education and Empowerment:** Many people living with neuropathy aren't aware of the full range of treatment options available to them. They may not know the right questions to ask or feel empowered to advocate for a more holistic approach to their care.

This combination of factors can create a perfect storm, leading to a healthcare system that often falls short in providing comprehensive and effective solutions for those suffering from neuropathy. However, by understanding these limitations and advocating for your own well-being, you can break free from this cycle and seek out a more empowering and holistic path to healing.

When Traditional Treatments Fall Short: Stories from the Frontlines of Neuropathy

While statistics paint a broad picture of any health condition, it's the individual stories—the real-life experiences of those living with neuropathy—that truly highlight the urgent need for a new approach. The following cases, documented in medical journals, illustrate the struggles many face with traditional neuropathy treatments and underscore the need for more effective, personalized solutions.

Case 1: A Teenager's Struggle with Treatment-Induced Neuropathy

Imagine being a 16-year-old just diagnosed with type 1 diabetes. You're starting treatment, hoping to regain control of your health, only to be hit with a new wave of challenges. This was the reality for a young girl who, just five weeks after beginning diabetes treatment, developed painful neuropathy in both feet, autonomic nervous system issues, and even vision problems (retinopathy) [2]. While her blood sugar levels improved significantly with treatment, her neuropathic symptoms persisted, highlighting how even successful management of an underlying condition doesn't always equate to neuropathy relief. Fortunately, after two months of dedicated care focused on symptom management, her neuropathy and retinopathy completely resolved. This case serves as a stark reminder that sometimes, the very treatments intended to help can inadvertently cause nerve damage, and that early recognition of such complications is crucial.

Case 2: The Challenge of Refractory Diabetic Peripheral Neuropathy

For some, diabetic neuropathy becomes a relentless adversary, resisting the effects of conventional treatments. This was the case for five individuals with refractory diabetic peripheral neuropathy (RDPN). These patients found no relief from standard therapies like blood sugar control medications and nutritional supplements [5]. Their pain persisted, highlighting a critical gap in traditional approaches. However, a glimmer of hope emerged when they were treated with a combination of ultrasound-guided hydrodissection—a minimally invasive procedure to release trapped nerves—and injections of mecobalamin, a form of vitamin B12 essential for nerve health. This innovative approach led to a noticeable reduction in pain and improvement in nerve function, underscoring the potential of exploring alternative therapies when conventional ones fail.

Case 3: Chronic Pain and the Limitations of First-Line Treatments

Traditional treatment for chronic neuropathic pain often involves a stepped approach, starting with medications like antidepressants and anticonvulsants. However, a review of multiple cases revealed that these first-line treatments often provide only partial or temporary relief, leaving patients grappling with persistent pain [3][4]. Despite trying various medications, many individuals continued to experience significant discomfort, highlighting the limitations of relying solely on pharmacological interventions. This led to the exploration of more advanced, interventional treatments like spinal cord stimulation and dorsal root ganglion stimulation. These approaches, while more invasive, offered better pain management for some, underscoring the need for a more comprehensive and individualized approach to chronic neuropathic pain.

Case 4: The Complexity of Post-Herpetic Neuralgia and Traumatic Nerve Injury

Post-herpetic neuralgia, a complication of shingles, and traumatic nerve injury are two common causes of neuropathic pain, often characterized by persistent, debilitating pain that standard treatments struggle to address [1]. In these cases, common medications like antidepressants and anticonvulsants often provide insufficient relief. Similarly, non-pharmacological interventions like cognitive behavioral therapy and hypnosis show limited effectiveness on their own. These cases underscore the need for a more integrated, multimodal approach to neuropathy care —one that combines medication, non-drug therapies, and personalized interventions to target the unique aspects of each individual's condition.

These are not just isolated cases; they represent a larger trend in neuropathy care where conventional approaches fall short of providing lasting relief. These stories underscore the critical need for innovative therapies like the WARRIOR Protocol—a holistic approach that addresses the root causes of neuropathy and empowers individuals to regain control of their health.

Citations:

[1] https://www.ncbi.nlm.nih.gov/pmc/articles/PMC9581623/

[2] https://www.ncbi.nlm.nih.gov/pmc/articles/PMC6790869/

[3] https://atm.amegroups.org/article/view/60475/html

[4] https://www.ncbi.nlm.nih.gov/pmc/articles/PMC6431761/

[5] https://www.frontiersin.org/journals/endocrinology/articles/10.3389/fendo.2021.735132/full

The WARRIOR Protocol: Your Personalized Path to Neuropathy Recovery

Imagine a treatment approach that doesn't just mask your symptoms but empowers your body to heal from the inside out. That's the driving force behind WARRIOR—a comprehensive, non-invasive program meticulously designed to address the root causes of neuropathy and restore your body's natural healing capabilities.

The WARRIOR Protocol is built on a simple yet powerful philosophy:

- **Address the Root Cause:** Instead of simply masking your symptoms, we focus on identifying and addressing the underlying factors contributing to your neuropathy. Whether it's blood sugar imbalances, inflammation, nutritional deficiencies, or nerve compression, we believe in treating the source, not just the symptoms.
- **Personalized Care:** No two cases of neuropathy are exactly alike. That's why we take a highly personalized approach, tailoring the WARRIOR Protocol to your unique needs, health history, and lifestyle factors.
- **Non-Invasive Therapies:** We believe in harnessing the body's innate healing abilities through safe, gentle, and non-invasive therapies. Our goal is to help you achieve lasting relief without relying on harsh medications or invasive procedures.

The Seven Pillars of W.A.R.R.I.O.R:

W – Water Hydration: Water is the lifeblood of your body, crucial for every cellular process, including nerve function. We help you optimize hydration, flushing out toxins, improving circulation, and supporting nerve health.

A – Anti-Inflammatory: Chronic inflammation is a silent saboteur, damaging nerves and hindering healing. The WARRIOR Protocol employs a multi-pronged attack on inflammation, incorporating dietary changes, targeted supplements, and therapies that calm the internal fire.

R – Revitalize Blood Flow: Like a vital supply line, healthy blood flow delivers essential oxygen and nutrients to your nerves. We utilize therapies that enhance circulation, revitalizing those crucial pathways and supporting nerve regeneration.

R – Restoration of Tissue Health: Neuropathy often involves damage to nerve tissues. The WARRIOR Protocol incorporates therapies specifically designed to promote tissue repair, stimulate cell regeneration, and restore the structural integrity of your nerves.

I – Improve Oxygenation: Oxygen is essential for cell health and regeneration, especially for energy-hungry nerves. We utilize techniques that enhance oxygen delivery, optimizing nerve function and accelerating the healing process.

O – Optimize Nutrition: Just as a warrior needs the right fuel for battle, your nerves rely on specific nutrients for optimal function and repair. We address potential deficiencies and provide personalized guidance to optimize your diet, ensuring your body has the building blocks for nerve health.

R – Rehabilitation & Functional Movement: Our ultimate goal is to help you regain your mobility, independence, and quality of life. The WARRIOR Protocol includes targeted exercises and therapies to strengthen weakened muscles, improve balance and coordination, and enhance your overall functional capacity, empowering you to return to the activities you love.

Premier Wellness Centers: Your Partner in Neuropathy Recovery

At Premier Wellness Centers, our chiropractic approach emphasizes the incredible healing capacity within every cell of your body, including your nerves. Our unique approach centers around three fundamental principles:

- **Oxygenation:** We utilize therapies that increase oxygen delivery to your cells, optimizing their function and accelerating the healing process.
- **Nutrition:** We work with you to identify potential nutrient deficiencies and develop personalized nutrition plans that provide

your body with the building blocks it needs for nerve regeneration and repair.

- **Stimulus-Driven Healing:** We utilize innovative therapies that gently stimulate your body's natural healing mechanisms, promoting nerve regeneration and restoring optimal function.

Our Comprehensive Approach Includes:

- **Hako-Med Electromedicine:** This innovative technology uses gentle electrical impulses to stimulate nerve regeneration, improve circulation, and reduce pain.
- **Infrared Light Therapy:** This safe and effective therapy uses specific wavelengths of light to reduce inflammation, improve blood flow, and stimulate cellular repair.
- **Vibration Therapy:** Gentle vibration therapy can enhance circulation, relax muscles, and improve nerve function.
- **Electrostimulation:** Targeted electrostimulation therapies can help re-educate muscles, improve coordination, and reduce pain.
- **SoftWave Therapy:** Our cutting-edge technology is proven to significantly decrease

inflammation and accelerate tissue regeneration, dramatically enhancing lives.

- **Targeted Supplementation:** We use a custom blend of pharmaceutical grade supplements to assist the body in reversing the metabolic drivers of the disease.
- **Paleo Diet:** Many healthy foods unfortunately can also support inflammatory responses in the body. We use a Paleo Low FODMAP diet to address these inflammatory drivers. .

Neuropathy Doesn't Define Me Anymore: Thanks to Premier Wellness Centers and the WARRIOR Protocol

"I highly recommend PWC. The staff is always warm and friendly. Dr. Jensen is knowledgeable and encouraging throughout your customized WARRIOR treatment plan. I am very grateful for overcoming issues with neuropathy that I had in my feet and legs."
- Cindy V.

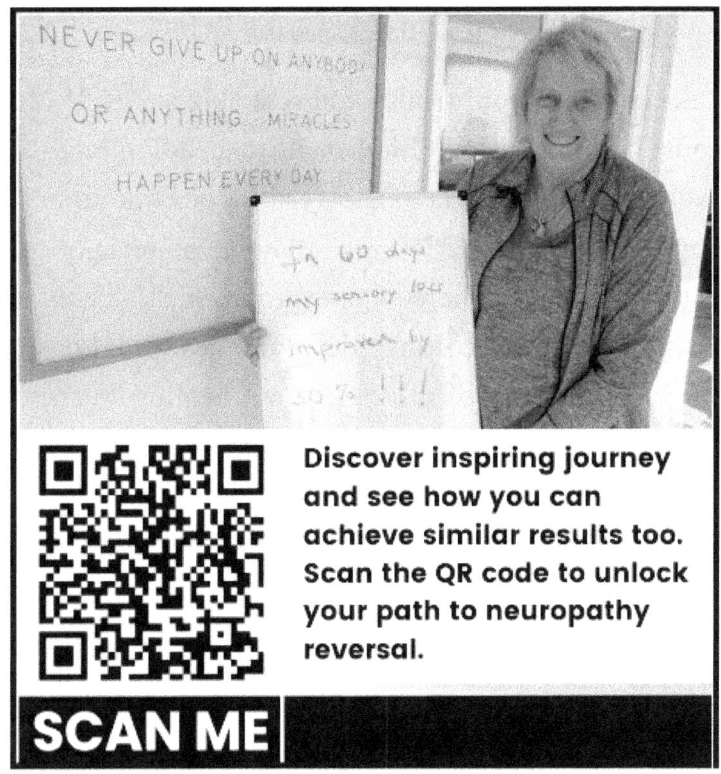

Unlock Your Path To Neuropathy Pain Relief Now: Call ((772) 279-4145 To Speak With A Caring Professional Today!

These testimonials reflect individual experiences and results, which may vary. They are not intended to represent or guarantee that everyone will achieve the same or similar outcomes.

Take the First Step Toward Lasting Relief

Take charge of your health and schedule a consultation with the chiropractic team at Premier Wellness Centers today. Discover how our unique approach to neuropathy care can help you reclaim your vitality. We're here to provide you with personalized care, cutting-edge therapies, and the support you need to embark on your healing journey. While we strive to offer the best possible care, a consultation does not guarantee specific results. Every individual's condition and response to treatment is unique.

 Unlock Your Path To Neuropathy Pain Relief Now: Call ((772) 279-4145 To Speak With A Caring Professional Today!

Individual results may vary. Please review the disclaimer after the Table of Contents.

3

SUGARCOATED SABOTAGE: UNRAVELING THE CONNECTION BETWEEN DIET, BLOOD SUGAR, AND NERVE HEALTH

John shuffled into my office, his shoulders slumped, his face etched with frustration. He'd been battling type 2 diabetes for years, diligently following his doctor's advice, taking his medications, and trying to make healthier choices. But despite his best efforts, the neuropathy in his feet just kept getting worse.

The burning pain was relentless, robbing him of sleep and making even simple tasks like walking the dog or standing to cook dinner excruciating. He felt trapped in a cycle of discomfort, his once-active lifestyle slowly slipping away.

When we discussed his diet, a familiar pattern emerged—a reliance on convenience foods, sugary drinks, and those all-too-common processed snacks that permeate the American diet. He knew these choices weren't ideal for his diabetes, but he hadn't realized the profound impact they were having on his neuropathy.

We worked together to create a personalized plan that focused on whole, unprocessed foods, emphasizing nutrient-dense meals that stabilized his blood sugar and reduced inflammation. He embraced the challenge, swapping processed snacks for fresh fruit and nuts, sugary drinks for water, and refined grains for fiber-rich alternatives.

The results were remarkable. Within weeks, the burning pain in his feet began to subside. His energy levels increased, his sleep improved, and a glimmer of hope returned to his eyes. He was able to take longer walks, engage in activities he'd given up on, and rediscover the joy of cooking healthy, delicious meals.

While we can't guarantee similar results for others, John's transformation highlights a powerful truth: the food we eat has a profound impact on our nerve health. By embracing a diet that nourishes our bodies instead of fueling inflammation and blood sugar imbalances, we can create a more healing environment from within, paving the way for neuropathy relief and lasting well-being.

This brings us to a crucial conversation about the typical American diet and its often-hidden role in contributing to neuropathy.

The American Diet: A Recipe for Neuropathy?

The American diet, sadly, is a whirlwind of convenience and indulgence. Processed foods, sugar-laden beverages, and an overreliance on refined grains have painted a landscape of potential health issues. This bombardment of "quick fixes" often comes at the expense of our well-being.

The nerve-wracking culprit in this food-fueled battle is sugar, disguised as a seemingly innocuous ingredient in a vast array of foods, from bread and sauces to yogurt. This covert sugar surge sends our blood sugar on a relentless roller coaster, leading to harmful peaks and crashes, impacting not only our physical health but also our fragile nervous system.

Imagine your nerves as delicate wires responsible for transmitting vital messages throughout your body. Now, picture those wires being coated in sticky syrup —that's essentially what happens when blood sugar levels remain consistently high. This "sugary sludge" interferes with nerve function, leading to those all-too-familiar symptoms of neuropathy: the tingling, numbness, pain, and loss of sensation.

It's not just about sugar. The way we eat, particularly our reliance on highly processed foods, plays a significant role in the neuropathy epidemic. Imagine taking a perfectly healthy piece of fruit, stripping it of its vital vitamins, and replacing them with artificial flavors and harmful additives. This is essentially what we're doing with many processed foods. The resulting inflammation sets off a chain reaction in our bodies, leaving our nerves weakened and struggling to heal.

It's time to face a difficult truth: the food choices we make every day can either nourish or harm our nerves. By understanding the link between diet, blood sugar, and nerve health, we can make informed choices to break free from this cycle of sugarcoated sabotage and reclaim our health, vitality, and well-being.

The Blood Sugar Rollercoaster: How Refined Carbs and Processed Foods Wreak Havoc on Your Nerves

Have you ever felt that sugar rush — a surge of energy that fizzles out as quickly as it arrived? This is a common reaction to consuming processed carbohydrates, which lack the complex fiber and nutrients found in whole foods. It's like giving your body a sugar shot without any sustainable fuel.

This roller coaster ride can wreak havoc on your blood sugar balance, forcing your pancreas into overdrive. The constant sugar spikes lead to a decline in insulin sensitivity, ultimately making your body resistant to its own powerful regulator. This resistance disrupts the delicate equilibrium of your blood sugar levels.

Processed foods further exacerbate this problem. They're often loaded with added sugars, unhealthy fats, and artificial ingredients that disrupt blood sugar balance and contribute to inflammation throughout the body. These foods are engineered for convenience and palatability, not for your body's long-term health.

This constant bombardment of sugar and refined carbohydrates keeps your body locked in a perpetual state of blood sugar dysregulation—a rollercoaster of highs and lows that takes a toll on your overall health, particularly your nerves. Over time, these blood sugar fluctuations damage the delicate blood vessels that supply nutrients and oxygen to your nerves. This damage disrupts nerve function, leading to the development and progression of neuropathy.

Nourishing Your Nerves: The Power of a Nutrient-Rich Diet

Just as a garden thrives on nutrient-rich soil, your nervous system relies on a steady supply of essential vitamins, minerals, and antioxidants to function optimally. When your diet lacks these vital nutrients, your nerves can become vulnerable to damage, leading to the development or worsening of neuropathy.

Think of your body as a complex machine, with each nutrient playing a specific role in keeping the gears turning smoothly. When it comes to nerve health, certain nutrients deserve special attention:

- **B Vitamins:** This family of vitamins, particularly B12, B6, and folate, are essential for nerve cell growth, repair, and the production of neurotransmitters—the chemical messengers that allow nerves to communicate with each other.
- **Vitamin D:** Often referred to as the "sunshine vitamin," vitamin D plays a crucial role in nerve cell growth and regeneration.
- **Magnesium:** This mighty mineral is involved in over 300 bodily processes, including nerve transmission, muscle function, and blood

sugar regulation—all of which are critical for maintaining healthy nerves.

- **Antioxidants:** These powerful compounds protect your cells from damage caused by free radicals, unstable molecules that can damage DNA and contribute to inflammation. Antioxidant-rich foods like berries, leafy greens, and nuts help shield your nerves from oxidative stress.
- **Omega-3 Fatty Acids:** Found in fatty fish like salmon and walnuts, these essential fats are vital components of nerve cell membranes, supporting their structure and function.

A diet rich in these and other essential nutrients provides the building blocks your body needs to maintain healthy nerves, repair damage, and reduce inflammation—all crucial for preventing and managing neuropathy.

When Food Choices Have Lasting Consequences: Real-Life Stories of Diet and Neuropathy

While we can talk about the science of nutrition and its impact on nerve health, sometimes, it's the human stories—the real-life experiences of those grappling with the consequences of dietary choices—that hit closest to home. Here are two cases that illustrate the very real link between the typical American diet, blood sugar imbalances, and the development of neuropathy.

Case 1: A Slow and Silent Onset of Neuropathy

Imagine being a 68-year-old man named C.T., enjoying your retirement years, only to be confronted with a gradual loss of sensation in your feet. C.T. had a history of impaired glucose tolerance, a condition often brought on by years of consuming a diet high in sugar and refined carbohydrates [1]. For six months, he'd noticed a tingling numbness in his feet, describing it as "walking on socks." While painless, this loss of sensation was concerning. After a thorough examination and nerve conduction study, C.T. was diagnosed with diabetic peripheral neuropathy. This case underscores the insidious nature of neuropathy; its onset can be gradual, and symptoms are often subtle in the early stages. It's a stark reminder that years of dietary choices that disrupt blood sugar can pave the way for nerve damage.

Case 2: Beyond Numbness: The Impact on Digestive Health

For some, the impact of high-sugar diets manifests not only in tingling limbs but also in severe digestive issues. One case, documented in *Diabetes Care,* tells the story of a man struggling with debilitating bouts of diarrhea, particularly at night, often accompanied by fecal incontinence [2]. He experienced a rollercoaster of digestive distress, enduring periods of frequent, watery bowel movements followed by days of constipation. This rollercoaster is characteristic of diabetic diarrhea, a condition distinct from other forms of diarrhea and often linked to nerve damage in the digestive system (diabetic enteropathy). This case serves as a stark reminder that the consequences of a diet high in sugar and processed foods can reach far beyond our waistlines, affecting vital systems throughout our bodies.

These cases illuminate a crucial point: The typical American diet, laden with refined carbohydrates, added sugars, and processed ingredients, sets the stage for blood sugar imbalances, paving the way for conditions like diabetes and its often-debilitating companion—neuropathy. These stories serve as a powerful call to action: By understanding the profound impact of our food choices, we can choose a different path—one that prioritizes nourishment, supports healthy blood sugar levels, and safeguards our precious nerve health.

Citations:

[1] https://diabetesjournals.org/clinical/article/19/3/122/
2461/Case-Study-A-68-Year-Old-Man-With-Diabetes-
and

[2] https://www.medicalnewstoday.com/articles/310937

The Gut-Nerve Connection: Unveiling a Surprising Link to Neuropathy

For years, we've viewed the gut and the brain as separate entities, each responsible for distinct functions. However, emerging research is revealing an intricate and fascinating connection between these two seemingly disparate systems – a link so profound that it's been dubbed the "gut-brain axis." What's more, this intricate connection extends to our nerves, playing a potential role in the development and progression of neuropathy.

You know how they say, "You are what you eat"? Well, it's even more complicated than that. There's a whole hidden world living inside your gut, a city of bacteria, fungi, and other microorganisms we call the gut microbiome. This bustling community impacts our health in surprising ways - from how we digest our food to our immunity and even our mental state.

And here's the fascinating part - recent discoveries link an imbalanced microbiome, or dysbiosis, to inflammation throughout the body, including our nervous system. Think of it like this: a bad neighborhood in the gut city can lead to an inflammatory fire, which can spread and damage our nerves, potentially worsening neuropathy.

Several factors can disrupt the delicate balance of our gut microbiome:

- **Diet:** A diet high in processed foods, sugar, and unhealthy fats can deplete beneficial gut bacteria, promoting the growth of harmful microbes that fuel inflammation.
- **Antibiotic Use:** While sometimes necessary, antibiotics can indiscriminately wipe out both good and bad bacteria in the gut, potentially leading to dysbiosis.
- **Stress:** Chronic stress can wreak havoc on our gut microbiome, disrupting its delicate balance and contributing to inflammation.
- **Underlying Health Conditions:** Certain health conditions, such as irritable bowel syndrome (IBS), inflammatory bowel disease (IBD), and autoimmune diseases, can also disrupt the gut microbiome and contribute to neuropathy.

This emerging understanding of the gut-nerve connection opens up exciting new possibilities for managing and relieving neuropathy. By nurturing a healthy gut microbiome through dietary changes, stress management techniques, and targeted probiotic supplementation, we can potentially reduce inflammation, protect our nerves, and support overall well-being.

It's a powerful fact: what we eat directly impacts our blood sugar and nerve health. Sadly, the typical American diet, loaded with sugary treats, refined grains, and processed meals, is a recipe for inflammation and nerve damage, leading to problems like neuropathy. But hold onto hope! We have the power to turn things around. By fueling our bodies with wholesome, nutrient-rich foods, we can stabilize blood sugar levels, creating an environment where our nerves can recover and flourish.

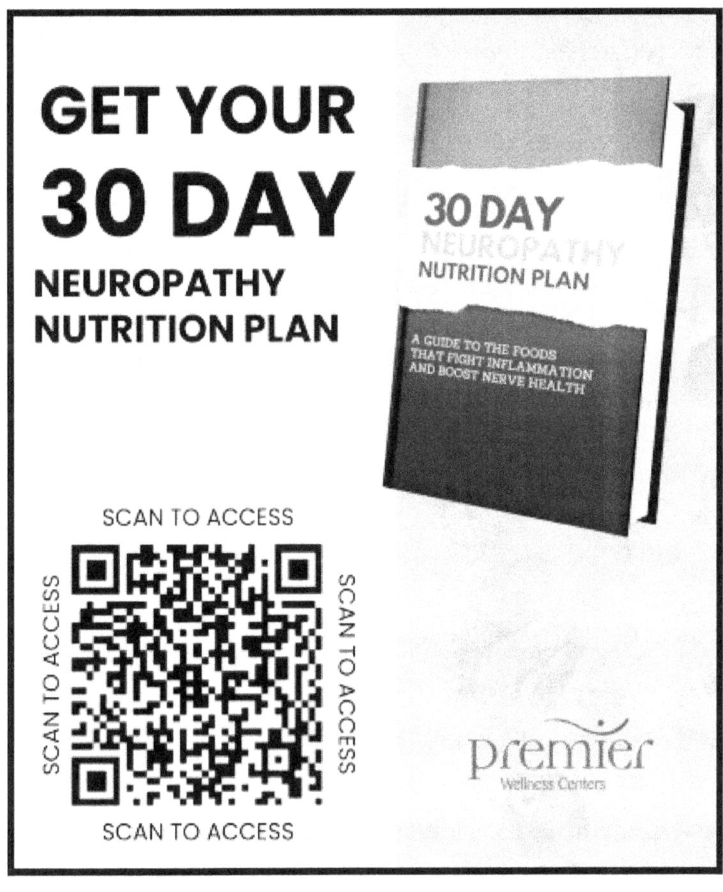

Unlock Your Path to Neuropathy Relief Now: Dial (772) 279-4145 to Speak With a Skilled Neuropathy Professional Today!

Individual results may vary. Please review the disclaimer after the Table of Contents.

4

———

THE INSULIN-NERVE CONNECTION: UNDERSTANDING THE KEY TO UNLOCKING NEUROPATHY RELIEF

Maria came to me with a look of quiet desperation. Prediabetes had cast a shadow over her life, and the early signs of neuropathy—that telltale tingling in her feet—had begun to chip away at her confidence. She was determined to prevent the progression to full-blown diabetes and the potential for debilitating nerve damage, but she felt lost in a maze of conflicting information and quick-fix promises.

We discussed the crucial role of insulin and blood sugar balance in preventing and managing neuropathy. I explained how the WARRIOR Protocol could help her body regain control of its blood sugar regulation, reduce inflammation, and support nerve health.

Maria embraced the program with a dedication that inspired me. She diligently followed her personalized dietary plan, incorporated regular exercise into her routine, and practiced stress management techniques. Week after week, I watched as her blood sugar levels stabilized, her energy increased, and the tingling in her feet gradually subsided.

Most importantly, a sense of empowerment returned to her eyes. She understood the intricate dance between insulin, glucagon, and blood sugar, and she had the tools to orchestrate that dance with grace and confidence. Maria's journey is a testament to the power of a holistic approach and the body's remarkable ability to heal when given the right support.

It's essential to note that results are not typical. Your experience may vary. However, Maria's story highlights a crucial point: by understanding the intricate mechanisms of blood sugar regulation and taking proactive steps to restore balance, we can create a more healing environment within our bodies, potentially preventing or relieving neuropathy.

This brings us to a deeper exploration of the intricate balancing act within our bodies.

The Balancing Act: How Insulin and Glucagon Orchestrate Blood Sugar Control

Imagine your body as a vast power grid, with glucose (sugar) as the essential energy source keeping everything running smoothly. Now, picture insulin and glucagon as two diligent workers, tirelessly maintaining the delicate balance of this energy grid. Insulin acts as the "storage manager," carefully ushering glucose from the bloodstream into your cells to be used for energy or stored for later use. Glucagon, on the other hand, serves as the "reserve power generator," releasing stored glucose into the bloodstream when energy levels run low.

This intricate dance between insulin and glucagon ensures that your body has a steady supply of energy, preventing those damaging highs and lows in blood sugar that can wreak havoc on your nerves. When this system functions optimally, your cells receive a constant flow of fuel, and your nerves can transmit messages without interference.

However, when this delicate balance is disrupted—as it often is in conditions like diabetes—nerve health can suffer. Chronically elevated blood sugar, whether from insufficient insulin production or cellular resistance to insulin's signals, creates a toxic environment for your nerves. Remember those delicate nerve fibers responsible for transmitting sensations and controlling muscle movements? They rely on a steady supply of oxygen and nutrients delivered through tiny blood vessels. High blood sugar damages these delicate vessels, essentially strangling the nerves and depriving them of essential nourishment.

Imagine trying to water a delicate plant with sugary soda instead of pure water. The plant wouldn't thrive; in fact, it would likely wither and die. The same principle applies to your nerves: chronically elevated blood sugar creates a similarly toxic environment, leading to nerve damage, dysfunction, and the often-debilitating symptoms of neuropathy.

This is why maintaining balanced blood sugar isn't just about preventing diabetes; it's crucial for protecting your nervous system and safeguarding your overall health and well-being.

The Unraveling: How Insulin Resistance Sets the Stage for Neuropathy

Insulin resistance is like a slow leak in a tire; it might not be noticeable at first, but over time, it can lead to a complete blowout. It's a progressive condition, often developing silently for years before any noticeable symptoms arise. And sadly, each stage of insulin resistance brings an increased risk of nerve damage and neuropathy.

Let's break down the stages and their connection to nerve health:

Stage 1: Early Insulin Resistance

In the early stages, your body starts producing more insulin to compensate for your cells' reduced sensitivity to its signals. You might not experience any noticeable symptoms, but behind the scenes, your pancreas is working overtime, and your cells are becoming less responsive to insulin's call to absorb glucose from the bloodstream.

Stage 2: Prediabetes

As insulin resistance progresses, your blood sugar levels start to rise, often exceeding the normal range. This is the prediabetes stage, a warning sign that your body is struggling to regulate blood sugar effectively. While you might not have neuropathy symptoms yet, this stage marks a critical turning point where nerve damage can begin.

Stage 3: Type 2 Diabetes

If insulin resistance remains unaddressed, it can progress to full-blown type 2 diabetes. At this stage, your blood sugar levels are consistently elevated, and the risk of nerve damage and neuropathy increases significantly. This is because the prolonged exposure to high blood sugar damages the delicate blood vessels that supply your nerves with oxygen and nutrients, leading to their dysfunction and degeneration.

The Vicious Cycle

Insulin resistance and neuropathy can feel like an unwelcome dance, each problem fueling the other. As nerve damage progresses, your body struggles to control blood sugar levels, amplifying insulin resistance. This creates a vicious cycle of escalating damage and increasing discomfort.

But hold onto hope – this cycle isn't destined to continue. By making positive changes in your lifestyle, from what you eat to how you manage stress, you can disrupt the domino effect and pave the way for healthier days.

Breaking Free: Lifestyle Strategies to Enhance Insulin Sensitivity and Protect Your Nerves

While the science behind insulin resistance and neuropathy might seem complex, the good news is that you have more power than you might realize to influence your metabolic health and protect your nerves. Simple yet profound lifestyle modifications can make a world of difference in improving insulin sensitivity, stabilizing blood sugar, and reducing your risk of nerve damage.

Think of these lifestyle changes not as quick fixes but as long-term investments in your health and well-being:

1. **Embrace a Blood-Sugar-Balancing Diet:** Your food choices have a direct and profound impact on your blood sugar levels and insulin sensitivity.

- **Prioritize Whole, Unprocessed Foods:** Focus on nutrient-dense foods like fruits, vegetables, whole grains, lean proteins, nuts, and seeds. These foods provide a steady stream of energy without causing dramatic spikes and crashes in blood sugar.
- **Limit Refined Carbs and Sugars:** Those sugary drinks, processed snacks, and refined

grains might offer a temporary energy boost, but they send your blood sugar on a roller coaster ride, wreaking havoc on your insulin sensitivity.

- **Embrace Healthy Fats:** Don't fear the fat! Healthy fats, found in foods like avocados, olive oil, nuts, and fatty fish, can actually improve insulin sensitivity and help stabilize blood sugar.

2. Make Movement Your Medicine: Physical activity isn't just about building muscles and burning calories; it's a potent way to enhance insulin sensitivity and improve your body's ability to utilize glucose effectively.

- **Find an Activity You Enjoy:** Whether it's brisk walking, dancing, swimming, cycling, or gardening, find a form of movement that you enjoy and can stick with long-term.
- **Aim for Consistency:** Even small amounts of movement throughout the day can make a difference. Take the stairs instead of the elevator, park farther away from your destination, or incorporate short walks into your routine.

3. Achieve and Maintain a Healthy Weight: Carrying excess weight, particularly around the abdomen, can increase inflammation and worsen insulin resistance.

- **Focus on Sustainable Changes:** Rather than resorting to crash diets, aim for gradual, sustainable changes to your eating habits and activity levels.
- **Celebrate Small Victories:** Every pound lost is a step in the right direction. Focus on progress, not perfection.

4. Prioritize Restful Sleep: Sleep deprivation not only leaves you feeling drained but also disrupts hormonal balance and can worsen insulin resistance.

- **Create a Relaxing Bedtime Routine:** Wind down an hour or two before bed by dimming the lights, taking a warm bath, reading, or practicing relaxation techniques.
- **Make Sleep a Non-Negotiable:** Aim for 7-9 hours of quality sleep each night.

5. Manage Stress Effectively: When you're stressed, your body releases hormones like cortisol, which can interfere with insulin's actions and increase blood sugar levels.

- **Incorporate Stress-Reducing Activities:** Explore activities that help you relax and unwind, such as yoga, meditation, deep breathing exercises, spending time in nature, or listening to calming music.
- **Seek Professional Support If Needed:** If you're struggling to manage stress on your own, don't hesitate to seek guidance from a therapist or counselor.

By making these lifestyle changes, you're not just improving insulin sensitivity and blood sugar control; you're creating a ripple effect of positive change throughout your body, supporting nerve health, reducing inflammation, and setting the stage for lasting well-being.

Exploring Additional Strategies for Blood Sugar Balance and Nerve Support

While lifestyle modifications form the cornerstone of improving insulin sensitivity and protecting nerve health, incorporating certain natural supplements can provide an extra layer of support. Think of these supplements as allies in your journey toward metabolic well-being:

1. Probiotics: Cultivating a Healthy Gut for Balanced Blood Sugar

As we've discussed, the gut microbiome plays a surprisingly crucial role in metabolic health. Probiotics, those beneficial bacteria that reside in our gut, can help improve insulin sensitivity, reduce inflammation, and potentially even protect against nerve damage.

- **How They Work:** Probiotics contribute to a healthy gut lining, which helps regulate the absorption of glucose into the bloodstream, preventing those damaging blood sugar spikes. They also help reduce inflammation throughout the body, including in the nervous system.
- **Food Sources:** Incorporate probiotic-rich foods into your diet, such as yogurt with live and active cultures, kefir, sauerkraut, kimchi, and miso.
- **Supplementation:** Consider a high-quality probiotic supplement to further support your gut health. Look for supplements that contain a variety of bacterial strains.

2. Berberine: A Natural Insulin Sensitizer

Berberine, a compound found in several plants, including goldenseal and barberry, has gained significant attention for its potential to improve blood sugar control and insulin sensitivity.

- **How It Works:** Berberine acts on multiple pathways involved in glucose metabolism, enhancing insulin sensitivity, reducing glucose production in the liver, and slowing down the absorption of carbohydrates in the gut.
- **Dosage and Considerations:** Dosage varies depending on individual needs and the form of berberine used. It's always best to consult with your healthcare provider before starting any new supplement, especially if you're taking other medications.

3. Cinnamon: Adding a Touch of Spice for Blood Sugar Control

This beloved spice isn't just for adding flavor to your favorite dishes; it also possesses blood-sugar-balancing properties that may benefit those with insulin resistance.

- **How It Works:** Cinnamon is believed to mimic the action of insulin, helping to usher glucose into cells more effectively. It may also slow down the breakdown of carbohydrates in the gut, leading to a more gradual rise in blood sugar after meals.
- **Ways to Incorporate:** Sprinkle cinnamon on your oatmeal, yogurt, or smoothies, or enjoy it in a warm cup of cinnamon tea.

4. Alpha-Lipoic Acid: A Powerful Antioxidant for Nerve Protection

Alpha-lipoic acid (ALA), a potent antioxidant, plays a vital role in cellular energy production and helps protect cells from oxidative stress—a key factor in nerve damage.

- **How It Works:** ALA acts as a potent free radical scavenger, neutralizing harmful molecules that can damage nerve cells. It also helps regenerate other antioxidants, including vitamin C and E, further boosting your body's defense system.
- **Food Sources:** ALA is found in small amounts in foods like spinach, broccoli, and organ meats.

- **Supplementation:** ALA supplements are available and may be beneficial for those with neuropathy, but it's always best to consult with your healthcare provider before starting any new supplement regimen.

Incorporating these additional strategies, in conjunction with lifestyle modifications, can create a synergistic approach to improve insulin sensitivity, protect your nerves, and support your overall metabolic health.

Understanding the intricate dance between insulin, glucagon, and blood sugar balance is like unlocking a crucial piece of the neuropathy puzzle. By addressing insulin resistance, we create a more stable internal environment where our nerves can thrive, not just survive. By embracing the power of lifestyle modifications and exploring evidence-based supplements, we empower ourselves to regain control of our metabolic health, paving the way for lasting relief from neuropathy and a brighter, healthier future.

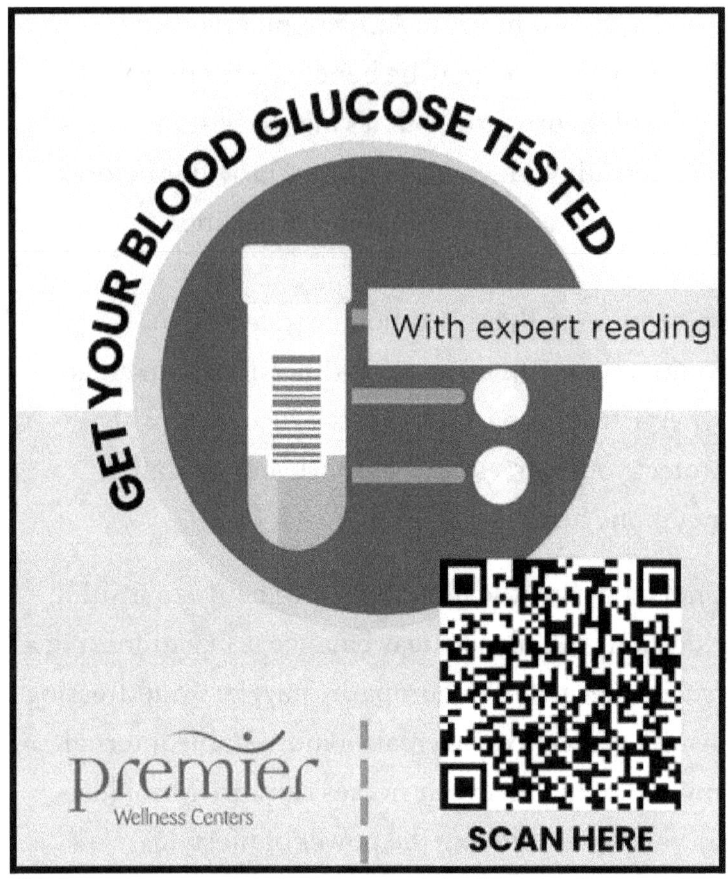

Unlock Your Path to Neuropathy Relief Now: Dial (772) 279-4145 to Speak With a Skilled Neuropathy Professional Today!

Individual results may vary. Please review the disclaimer after the Table of Contents.

5

IGNITE YOUR INNER HEALER: NATURAL THERAPIES TO RELIEVE NEUROPATHY

Lisa arrived at my office with a heavy heart and a weary body. Neuropathy had woven its way into her life, leaving her hands numb, her feet burning, and her spirit dimmed. She'd tried various medications, physical therapy, and even acupuncture, but the relief was always temporary, never addressing the root of her suffering. She felt like she was simply managing symptoms, not truly healing.

I introduced her to the philosophy behind the WARRIOR Protocol—a holistic approach that views the body as an interconnected system, acknowledging the interplay of physical, emotional, and lifestyle factors in the development and progression of neuropathy.

Lisa embraced this holistic approach with an open mind and a determined spirit. She adopted the anti-inflammatory diet we discussed, replacing processed foods with vibrant, nutrient-rich meals. She began incorporating gentle yoga and meditation into her daily routine, finding solace in movement and stillness. And she committed to addressing the emotional stress that had been weighing heavily on her.

The transformation was remarkable. The numbness in her hands gradually lessened, the burning in her feet subsided, and her energy returned. Most importantly, a sense of vitality, a spark of joy, re-emerged in her eyes. It wasn't just about symptom relief; it was about rediscovering a sense of wholeness, of vibrant well-being that radiated from within.

This is one individual's experience and does not guarantee similar results. However, Lisa's journey highlights a crucial point: true healing extends far beyond simply addressing physical symptoms.

The Holistic Approach: Shifting from Symptom Management to Whole-Body Healing

Neuropathy has traditionally been managed by suppressing symptoms—masking pain, reducing tingling, and limiting the impact on daily life.

However, what if we could go beyond symptom control and target the underlying causes? A holistic approach to neuropathy emphasizes restoring balance within the body's intricate systems to awaken its innate healing capabilities.

Consider your body as an orchestrated system of interconnected elements. Each component, from cells to organs, is crucial in maintaining overall well-being. Neuropathy often signals a disruption within this intricate balance, potentially arising from factors such as insufficient nutrient delivery to nerves, persistent inflammation, or fluctuating blood sugar levels. A holistic approach addresses these imbalances, fine-tuning your body's inner symphony for lasting health and recovery.

Fueling Resilience: A Dietary Approach to Preventing Neuropathy

Food isn't just calories on a plate; it's a powerful medicine that can either fuel disease or nourish your body back to health. By making conscious food choices, you can create an internal environment that supports nerve health, reduces inflammation, and enhances your body's ability to heal.

Embrace the Power of Whole Foods:

- **Low-Glycemic:** As we've discussed, stabilizing blood sugar is paramount for nerve health. Embrace a low-glycemic diet that emphasizes foods that have a minimal impact on blood sugar levels, such as non-starchy vegetables, low-sugar fruits, lean proteins, and healthy fats.

- **Anti-Inflammatory:** Imagine dousing a fire with water instead of gasoline. That's the power of an anti-inflammatory diet. Load up on foods rich in antioxidants and omega-3 fatty acids—think colorful vegetables, berries, fatty fish, nuts, and seeds—to help calm the flames of inflammation that contribute to nerve damage.

- **Nutrient-Dense:** Your nerves rely on a steady supply of specific vitamins, minerals, and antioxidants to function optimally. Fuel them with a diet rich in colorful fruits and vegetables, leafy greens, nuts, seeds, and lean proteins.

Key Dietary Allies for Nerve Health:

- **Fiber:** This indigestible plant matter acts like a broom in your digestive tract, slowing down sugar absorption and promoting stable blood sugar levels. It also supports a healthy gut microbiome—an often-overlooked factor in nerve health.

- **Healthy Fats:** Don't fear the fat! Healthy fats, found in avocados, olive oil, nuts, and fatty fish, are crucial for nerve cell structure and function. They also help reduce inflammation and support blood sugar balance.

- **Antioxidants:** These powerful compounds act like bodyguards for your cells, protecting them from damage caused by free radicals— unstable molecules that contribute to inflammation and nerve damage.

By adopting a holistic approach to neuropathy that prioritizes a nutrient-rich, blood-sugar-balancing, and anti-inflammatory diet, you're not just managing symptoms; you're empowering your body's innate healing abilities and creating a foundation for lasting relief and optimal health.

Food as Medicine: Witnessing the Transformative Power of Dietary Change

When you consistently nourish your body with the right foods, you're not just providing fuel; you're initiating a cascade of positive changes that ripple through your entire system, transforming your health from the inside out. Here's how a shift towards a healing diet can specifically impact those struggling with neuropathy:

Taming the Flames: Reducing Inflammation for Nerve Healing

Inflammation is often described as a "necessary evil." It's your body's natural response to injury or infection, a way of protecting and healing itself. However, when inflammation becomes chronic—like a fire alarm that never shuts off—it can cause more harm than good, contributing to a wide range of health problems, including neuropathy.

A diet rich in anti-inflammatory foods can help calm this internal fire, creating an environment where your nerves can begin to heal. By reducing inflammation, you're essentially clearing the debris and creating a fertile ground for nerve regeneration.

Balancing the Scales: The Power of Stable Blood Sugar

We've already established the damaging effects of blood sugar spikes and crashes on your nerves. By adopting a low-glycemic diet, you're effectively taking control of your body's energy supply, ensuring a steady and sustainable stream of fuel without the damaging fluctuations that can harm your nerves.

Imagine driving a car with a jerky accelerator, constantly hitting the gas and then slamming on the brakes. It wouldn't be a smooth ride, would it? Your body functions similarly. Stable blood sugar promotes smoother operations throughout your system, reducing stress on your nerves and allowing them to function optimally.

Filling the Gaps: Replenishing Vital Nutrients for Nerve Health

Often, neuropathy develops or worsens due to nutritional deficiencies. Your nerves require a specific blend of vitamins, minerals, and antioxidants to function properly. By embracing a nutrient-dense diet, you're providing your body with the building blocks it needs to repair damaged nerves, protect healthy ones, and optimize nerve communication.

This nutritional replenishment is like providing your body with a skilled construction crew and high-quality materials to repair a damaged bridge. With the right resources, your body can begin the work of rebuilding and restoring those crucial nerve pathways.

This isn't just about alleviating symptoms; it's about addressing the root causes of neuropathy and fostering a state of vibrant well-being from within. It's about empowering your body to heal itself—naturally and effectively.

Putting It Into Practice: Your Delicious Guide to Nerve-Nourishing Meals

You now understand the "why" behind a nerve-healthy diet, but you might be wondering, "What does that actually look like on my plate?" Fear not! We're about to translate nutritional science into delicious, satisfying meals that nourish your body and support your journey toward neuropathy relief.

Remember, this is not about deprivation or complicated recipes. It's about making simple, sustainable changes that bring joy back to mealtime while providing your body with the nutrients it needs to thrive.

A Sample Day of Nerve-Nourishing Deliciousness

Here's a glimpse into what a day of eating for nerve health might look like:

- **Breakfast:** Start your day with a blood-sugar-balancing breakfast that provides sustained energy:

- **Option 1:** Scrambled eggs with spinach and a side of berries
  - **Option 2:** Chia seed pudding topped with almonds and blueberries
  - **Option 3:** Smoothie made with unsweetened almond milk, spinach, berries, and a scoop of protein powder.
- **Lunch:** Keep your energy levels stable and nourish your nerves with these lunch ideas:
  - **Option 1:** Large salad with grilled chicken or fish, avocado, a variety of colorful vegetables, and a light vinaigrette dressing.
  - **Option 2:** Lentil soup with a side of sourdough bread and a mixed green salad.
  - **Option 3:** Leftovers from dinner!
- **Dinner:** End your day with a delicious and satisfying meal that supports nerve health:
  - **Option 1:** Baked salmon with roasted green beans and white rice.
  - **Option 2:** Chicken and vegetable stir-fry served over white potatoes.
  - **Option 3:** Turkey meatballs with zucchini noodles and garlic infused oil..

Snacks: Keep healthy snacks on hand to prevent blood sugar dips and nourish your body between meals:

- A handful of pistachios or walnuts
- A piece of fruit with a tablespoon of nut butter
- Carrot sticks or celery sticks with hummus
- Coconut yogurt with berries and a sprinkle of cinnamon

Recipe Inspiration: Turmeric-Roasted Chickpeas

These crunchy, flavorful chickpeas are packed with protein, fiber, and anti-inflammatory spices. Enjoy them as a snack, salad topper, or side dish.

Ingredients:

- 1 can (15 ounces) canned chickpeas, rinsed and drained
- 1 tablespoon olive oil
- 1 teaspoon turmeric
- 1/2 teaspoon cumin
- 1/4 teaspoon sea salt

Instructions:

1. Preheat oven to 400 degrees F (200 degrees C).
2. Toss chickpeas with olive oil, turmeric, cumin, and salt on a baking sheet.
3. Roast for 20-25 minutes, or until crispy, stirring halfway through.

Remember, this is just a starting point. There are endless possibilities to create delicious and nourishing meals that support your neuropathy healing journey!

Get Moving for Nerve Health: Unleashing the Power of Exercise

When it comes to managing neuropathy, exercise might not be the first thing that springs to mind. You might even be thinking, "Exercise? But my feet tingle, my legs feel weak, and I'm in pain!" While it's crucial to listen to your body and avoid any movements that exacerbate your symptoms, embracing a safe and appropriate exercise routine can be surprisingly transformative for neuropathy.

Think of exercise as a gentle wake-up call for your nerves, encouraging them to regenerate, reconnect, and function more effectively. Here's how regular movement can make a difference:

- **Enhanced Nerve Function:** Just like a muscle that gets stronger with use, your nerves can benefit from regular activity. Exercise stimulates nerve regeneration, promotes the growth of new nerve endings, and helps re-establish those crucial pathways that transmit signals throughout your body.

- **Improved Strength and Flexibility:** Neuropathy often leads to muscle weakness and stiffness, making everyday movements challenging. Exercise helps combat these effects by strengthening muscles, improving flexibility, and enhancing your range of motion. This can make it easier to maintain your balance, walk with greater confidence, and perform daily tasks with greater ease.

- **Boosted Circulation:** Remember those tiny blood vessels responsible for delivering oxygen and nutrients to your nerves? Exercise is like a pump for your circulatory system, improving blood flow throughout your body, including to those often-compromised nerves. This enhanced circulation delivers vital nourishment to your nerves, promoting their repair and regeneration.

- **Overall Well-Being Boost:** Exercise isn't just good for your body; it does wonders for your mind and spirit too. It releases endorphins—those feel-good chemicals that act as natural pain relievers—helping to lift your mood, reduce stress, and improve sleep quality.

The key is to start slowly, listen to your body, and choose activities appropriate for your fitness level and the severity of your neuropathy.

Finding Your Move: Effective Exercise Options for Neuropathy

Now that you understand the remarkable benefits of exercise for neuropathy, let's explore some specific activities that can make a real difference in your journey toward greater strength, mobility, and nerve health:

1. Find Your Footing: Balance and Gait Training

Neuropathy often affects our sense of balance and coordination, increasing the risk of falls. Balance and gait training exercises help retrain your brain and body to work together seamlessly, improving stability and confidence.

- **Simple Exercises:** Start with simple exercises like standing on one leg, walking heel-to-toe in a straight line, or practicing gentle tai chi movements.
- **Increase Challenge Gradually:** As your balance improves, you can increase the challenge by incorporating activities like yoga or Pilates, which challenge your balance and coordination in dynamic ways.

2. Get Your Heart Pumping: Aerobic Exercise

Aerobic exercise not only strengthens your heart and lungs but also enhances blood flow throughout your body, delivering vital oxygen and nutrients to your nerves.

- **Low-Impact Options:** Choose low-impact activities like walking, swimming, water aerobics, or cycling, which are gentler on your joints.
- **Start Slowly:** Begin with short sessions and gradually increase the duration and intensity as your fitness improves.

3. Build Strength and Resilience: Strength Training

Strength training helps build muscle mass, which is crucial for supporting and protecting your joints, improving balance, and enhancing overall mobility.

- **Bodyweight Exercises:** Start with bodyweight exercises like squats, lunges, push-ups, and wall sits.
- **Resistance Bands or Light Weights:** As you gain strength, you can incorporate resistance bands or light weights to further challenge your muscles.

4. Enhance Flexibility and Range of Motion: Stretching

Regular stretching helps improve flexibility, reduce muscle stiffness, and prevent injuries. It can also help alleviate those tight, constricted feelings often associated with neuropathy.

- **Gentle Stretches:** Focus on gentle stretches that target the muscles in your legs, feet, and hands—areas often affected by neuropathy.
- **Yoga or Pilates:** These practices incorporate a beautiful blend of strength training,

flexibility, and balance work, making them excellent choices for those with neuropathy.

5. Water Workouts: The Power of Buoyancy

Exercising in water provides gentle resistance and buoyancy, supporting your joints, reducing the risk of injury, and making movement more comfortable.

- **Water Aerobics or Swimming:** These activities provide a full-body workout without putting excessive stress on your joints.
- **Water Walking or Running:** Even simply walking or jogging in water can be beneficial, providing resistance and support.

Consistency is key! Aim for at least 30 minutes of moderate-intensity exercise most days of the week. Always listen to your body, start slowly, and gradually increase the intensity and duration of your workouts as your fitness improves.

Finding Calm Amidst the Storm: The Profound Impact of Stress Management on Neuropathy

Did you know stress can actually harm your nerves? Think of your stress response as a life raft in an emergency. It helps you overcome challenging situations by boosting your energy with a surge of adrenaline and cortisol. However, in today's fast-paced world, many of us live in a constant state of stress. The endless flow of demands, deadlines, and digital overload leaves our stress response perpetually on high alert. This constant pumping of adrenaline and cortisol can take a toll on our delicate nervous system, like a garden left unkempt eventually turning overgrown and neglected.

Here's how chronic stress can exacerbate neuropathy:

- **Hormonal Havoc:** Remember cortisol, that stress hormone designed to help us cope with acute threats? When cortisol levels remain chronically elevated, it can interfere with blood sugar regulation, increase inflammation throughout the body, and even damage nerve cells directly.
- **Amplified Pain Perception:** Stress has a sneaky way of turning up the volume on pain signals. When you're stressed, your body is in a heightened state of alert, making you more sensitive to pain and discomfort.
- **Sleep Disruption:** Stress and sleep are like oil and water—they simply don't mix. When you're chronically stressed, it can be

challenging to quiet your mind and achieve restful sleep. This lack of sleep further disrupts hormonal balance, increases inflammation, and hinders your body's ability to repair and regenerate, including nerve cells.

- **Immune System Suppression:** Chronic stress weakens your immune system, making you more susceptible to infections that can further damage nerves.

This intricate connection between stress and neuropathy highlights a crucial point: managing stress isn't just about improving your mood; it's an essential component of protecting your nerve health and supporting your overall well-being.

Cultivating Calm: Your Toolkit for Effective Stress Management

You wouldn't ignore a smoke alarm blaring in your home, would you? Chronic stress is your body's way of signaling that something is out of balance. It's a call to take action, to incorporate practices that soothe your nervous system, quiet your mind, and restore a sense of calm amidst life's inevitable storms.

The good news is that you have a wealth of tools at

your disposal to effectively manage stress and protect your precious nerve health:

1. Tap Into the Power of the Present Moment: Mindfulness and Meditation

Mindfulness isn't about emptying your mind or pretending negative feelings don't exist – it's about simply acknowledging what's going on without getting carried away. Think of it as being present without judgment – noticing the thoughts flitting through your mind, the feelings you're experiencing, and even the sensations in your body, without clinging to them or letting them control you. Meditation is a tool for cultivating mindfulness. It invites you to anchor your attention on something specific – your breath, a mantra, or even a gentle visual—to quiet the chatter in your head and bring about a state of peaceful awareness.

- **Start Small:** Begin with just a few minutes of mindfulness or meditation each day, gradually increasing the duration as you become more comfortable.
- **Guided Meditations:** Explore guided meditations specifically designed for stress reduction, pain management, or sleep improvement.

2. Strike a Pose for Calm: Yoga

Yoga is a beautiful blend of physical postures, controlled breathing, and meditation that calms the nervous system, reduces stress hormones, and promotes relaxation.

- **Gentle Styles:** Explore gentle styles like restorative yoga or yin yoga, which focus on holding poses for extended periods to promote deep relaxation.
- **Chair Yoga:** If mobility is a challenge, try chair yoga, a gentle form of yoga that can be done sitting or using a chair for support.

3. Breathe Your Way to Calm: Deep Breathing Exercises

Deep, diaphragmatic breathing is like a reset button for your nervous system. It helps slow your heart rate, lower blood pressure, and ease muscle tension.

- **Try the 4-7-8 Technique:** Inhale deeply through your nose for a count of 4, hold your breath for a count of 7, and exhale slowly through your mouth for a count of 8. Repeat for several rounds.

- **Practice Anytime, Anywhere:** Incorporate deep breathing exercises into your daily routine—while driving, working at your desk, or before bed.

4. Relax from Head to Toe: Progressive Muscle Relaxation

Progressive muscle relaxation (PMR) involves systematically tensing and relaxing different muscle groups in your body. This technique helps you become more aware of muscle tension and promotes deep relaxation.

- **Guided Practice:** Find guided PMR exercises online or through smartphone apps.
- **Incorporate Into Daily Life:** Practice PMR before bed, during stressful situations, or anytime you need to unwind.

5. Harness the Power of Biofeedback:

Biofeedback uses sensors to monitor physiological processes like muscle tension, heart rate, and skin temperature, providing you with real-time feedback on your body's stress response.

- **Learn to Control Your Body's Responses:** With practice, you can learn to consciously control these functions, reducing stress and promoting relaxation.
- **Seek Professional Guidance:** Biofeedback is typically conducted with a trained therapist.

6. Reconnect with Nature:

Nature has a remarkable ability to soothe our souls and quiet our minds. Spending time outdoors, even for a few minutes each day, can have a profound impact on stress levels.

- **Take a Walk in the Park:** Immerse yourself in the sights, sounds, and smells of nature.
- **Grounding Techniques:** Try grounding techniques, like walking barefoot on grass or sand, to feel more connected to the earth.

7. Nurture Your Social Connections:

Strong social connections provide a buffer against stress and offer a source of support during challenging times.

- **Make Time for Loved Ones:** Prioritize quality time with family and friends.

- **Join a Group or Club:** Engage in activities you enjoy and connect with others who share your interests.

8. Engage in Activities You Enjoy:

Hobbies and activities you love provide a much-needed respite from stress and allow you to tap into your passions.

- **Schedule Time for Fun:** Make time for activities that bring you joy, whether it's reading, painting, gardening, listening to music, or spending time with loved ones.

Managing stress is an ongoing journey, not a destination. Experiment with different techniques to find what works best for you and incorporate them into your daily life to create a more peaceful, resilient, and nerve-healthy you.

Making It Happen: Weaving Stress Management into Your Daily Life

You now have a toolbox filled with powerful stress management techniques, but you might be wondering, "How do I actually fit these into my already busy life?" The key is to start small, be patient with yourself, and view stress management not as another task on your to-do list but as an investment in your overall well-being.

Here are a few tips to seamlessly integrate these practices into your daily routine:

- **Start with Just 5 Minutes:** You don't have to become a meditation master overnight. Begin with just 5 minutes of deep breathing or a guided meditation each day and gradually increase the duration as you feel comfortable.
- **Link It to an Existing Habit:** Make it easier to remember by linking your chosen stress management technique to an existing habit. For example, practice deep breathing while you're waiting for your morning coffee to brew or listen to a guided meditation while you're commuting.
- **Schedule It In:** Just as you schedule important appointments and meetings, block out time in your day for stress-reducing activities. Treat these appointments with the same level of importance as any other commitment.
- **Transform Everyday Moments:** Look for opportunities to incorporate mindfulness into everyday tasks. Pay attention to your

senses while you're eating, walking, showering, or washing dishes.

- **Create a Soothing Bedtime Routine:** Wind down an hour or two before bed with relaxing activities like taking a warm bath, reading, or gentle stretching. Avoid screen time during this time, as the blue light emitted from electronic devices can interfere with melatonin production, a hormone essential for sleep.
- **Be Kind to Yourself:** There will be days when you miss a meditation session or find yourself feeling more stressed than usual. That's okay. Don't beat yourself up. Simply acknowledge it and gently guide yourself back to your chosen stress management practices.

Remember, it's about progress, not perfection. It's about making small, consistent choices each day to nurture your nervous system, cultivate inner peace, and support your overall health and well-being.

We've learned that healing is a much deeper process than just fixing what's broken. It's about caring for our entire selves – nourishing our bodies, calming our minds, and feeding our spirits. Imagine unleashing your body's hidden healing power through wholesome food, regular movement, and finding ways to conquer stress. By embracing this holistic approach, neuropathy might not feel like an insurmountable hurdle. Instead, it becomes a turning point on a path toward lasting relief, vibrant health, and a life overflowing with energy, peace, and happiness.

ACTION STEP: Get Your Neuropathy Relief Stretch Handbook. **Master 11 Key Stretches** from Home To *Retrain Your Nerves and Regain Your Life.*

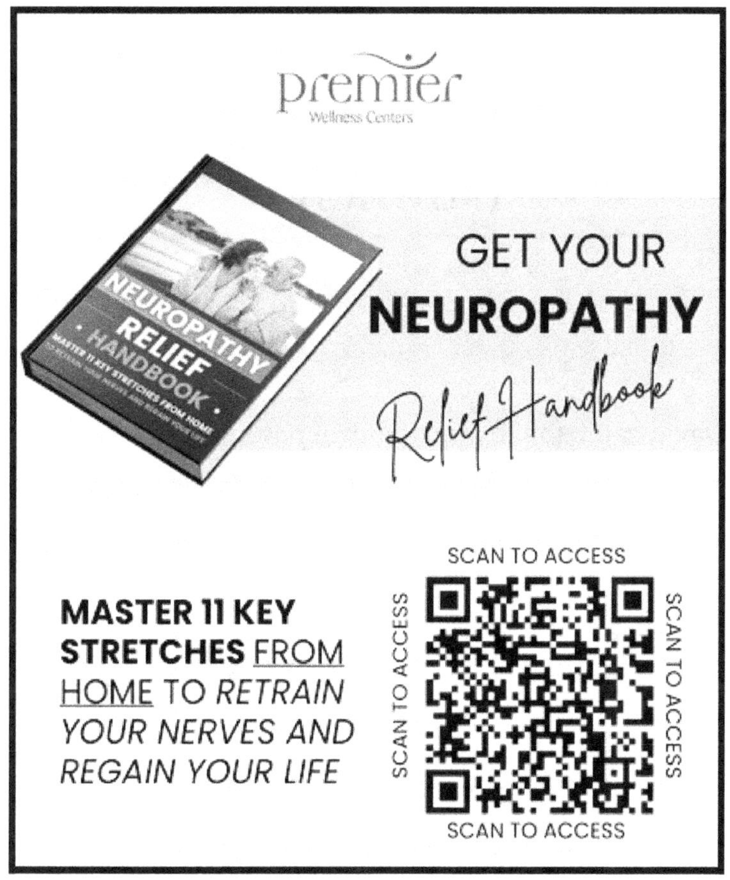

Unlock Your Path to Neuropathy Relief Now: Dial (772) 279-4145 to Speak With a Skilled Neuropathy Professional Today!

6

BEWARE OF FALSE PROMISES: SEPARATING NEUROPATHY FACT FROM FICTION

David came to me after years of battling peripheral neuropathy. He'd been down the road of countless quick fixes—expensive supplements, topical creams, even experimental devices—each promising to be the miracle cure he desperately sought. But each time, hope turned to disappointment as the tingling and numbness persisted, the pain returned, and his frustration grew.

He was skeptical when I explained the WARRIOR Protocol—a comprehensive approach that focused on addressing the root causes of his neuropathy, not just masking the symptoms. It wasn't a quick fix; it required commitment, lifestyle changes, and a willingness to embrace a holistic approach to healing.

But David was tired of chasing empty promises. He was ready for a real solution. He committed to the program, attending his therapy sessions diligently, making dietary changes, incorporating gentle exercise into his routine, and learning to manage stress more effectively.

It wasn't an overnight miracle, but gradually, David began to experience lasting relief. The tingling subsided, the numbness lessened, and the pain became manageable. He regained strength and stability, rediscovering the joy of activities he'd long given up on.

David's story is a powerful reminder that true healing rarely comes in a bottle or a quick fix. It's essential to remember that individual outcomes may differ. However, his journey highlights the importance of addressing the root causes of neuropathy, embracing a holistic approach, and making sustainable lifestyle changes.

This brings us to a crucial conversation about the allure—and often the deception—of quick fixes for neuropathy.

The Allure (and Deception) of Quick Fixes

Living with neuropathy means battling a relentless tide of symptoms. It's a struggle for anyone to endure the tingling, burning, and numbness, making you crave a solution - and quickly. This longing for a quick fix, however, makes you vulnerable to the misinformation readily available online.

From self-proclaimed miracle cures to the "natural" remedy of the day, the internet can easily mislead you with its promises of immediate relief. While hope is essential, relying on proven medical advice and treatments remains paramount. Talk to your doctor and work together to navigate the complexities of neuropathy. Don't fall for dubious claims – trust the expertise of those who truly understand your condition.

Why Home Remedies Often Miss the Mark

Many home remedies, while well-intentioned, simply aren't designed to address the complex underlying causes of neuropathy. They might provide temporary relief from symptoms, but they rarely address the root of the problem.

Think of it this way: imagine trying to fix a cracked foundation in your home by simply painting over the cracks. While the fresh paint might conceal the problem temporarily, it does nothing to address the underlying structural damage. Similarly, applying a topical cream or soaking your feet in Epsom salts might offer temporary relief from neuropathy symptoms, but it won't address the underlying nerve damage or the factors that caused it.

Moreover, some home remedies can actually be harmful, especially if they involve using substances not intended for medicinal use or if they lead you to delay seeking proper medical care. It's also important to consider the financial costs associated with chasing after numerous remedies that offer little to no benefit. Those seemingly inexpensive ingredients can add up over time, leaving your wallet lighter and your neuropathy no better.

Navigating the Supplement Maze: Separating Hype from True Healing

While the world of supplements can be alluring, with promises of easy solutions for nerve health issues, the truth is that this market often lacks reliable guidance and regulation. This means the actual contents and efficacy of many supplements haven't been rigorously proven. Always exercise caution and seek scientific validation before choosing any supplement. Be an informed consumer; understand the potential risks and rewards of supplementation before adding them to your routine.

Take vitamin B6, for example. It's essential for nerve health, and a deficiency can certainly contribute to neuropathy. However, vitamin B6 comes in various forms, some beneficial and others potentially harmful in high doses. Pyridoxine, a common form of B6 found in many supplements, can actually worsen nerve damage if taken in excessive amounts. This highlights the crucial need for informed guidance when choosing supplements, as more isn't always better.

Even seemingly harmless supplements can have unintended consequences:

- **Drug Interactions:** Supplements can interact with medications, potentially interfering with their effectiveness or causing adverse side effects.
- **Allergic Reactions:** Some individuals may have allergies or sensitivities to certain ingredients commonly found in supplements.
- **Digestive Upset:** Supplements, particularly those taken in high doses or on an empty

stomach, can cause digestive upset, including nausea, diarrhea, or constipation.

This isn't to say that all supplements are ineffective or dangerous; some can be valuable allies in your neuropathy healing journey. However, it's crucial to approach supplementation with a discerning eye and always consult with your healthcare provider before adding anything new to your regimen, especially if you're taking other medications.

While research is ongoing, and individual responses to supplements can vary, some supplements have shown promise in supporting nerve health:

- **L-Citrulline:** This amino acid helps increase nitric oxide production, which relaxes blood vessels and improves circulation—a crucial factor in supporting nerve health.
- **L-Glutathione:** Often referred to as the "master antioxidant," glutathione helps protect cells from oxidative stress, a key contributor to nerve damage.
- **Vitamin B12:** A deficiency in vitamin B12 is a known cause of neuropathy. Supplementation can be particularly beneficial for those with absorption issues or dietary deficiencies.

- **Acetyl-L-Carnitine:** This amino acid plays a vital role in nerve cell energy production and has shown some promise in improving nerve function in those with neuropathy.
- **Alpha-Lipoic Acid (ALA):** As a potent antioxidant, ALA helps protect nerves from oxidative damage and may promote nerve regeneration.
- **Amarasate:** Derived from spinach, this compound may help protect nerve cells from damage and reduce inflammation.

Remember, supplements aren't a quick fix for neuropathy. They work best within a comprehensive chiropractic approach at Premier Wellness Centers that addresses root causes, encourages lifestyle modifications, and involves close collaboration with your chiropractor. We can assess your individual needs and advise on appropriate supplements aligned with your health goals and overall treatment plan.

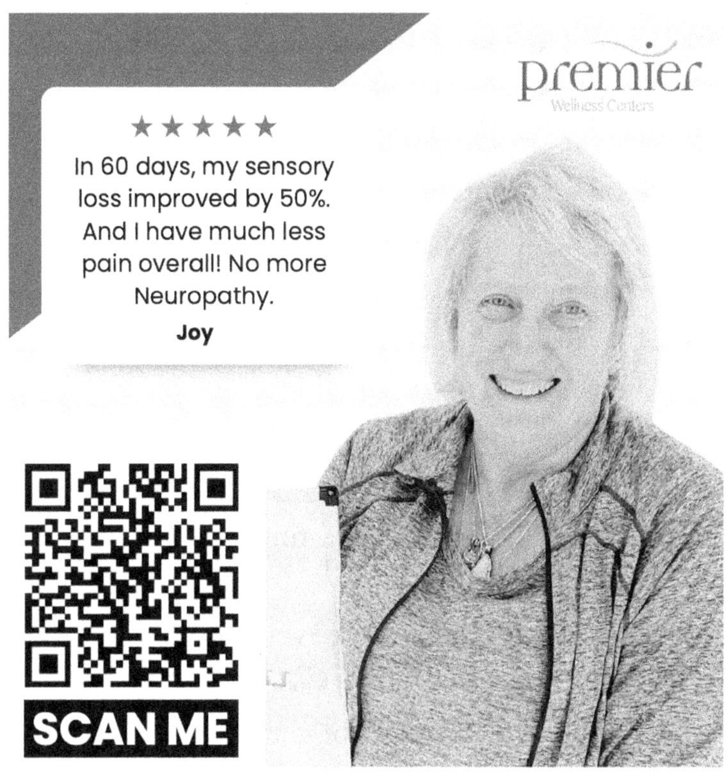

The High Cost of Quick Fixes: Why They Set You Up for Disappointment

The allure of a quick fix is powerful, especially when you're in pain and desperate for relief. But when it comes to complex conditions like neuropathy, those promises of rapid results often come with hidden costs—to your health, your wallet, and your overall well-being.

Here's why those quick-fix promises often fall flat:

- **Lack of Scientific Rigor:** Many quick fixes for neuropathy lack rigorous scientific evidence to support their claims. They might be based on anecdotal evidence, testimonials, or outdated theories that haven't stood the test of time.

- **Unrealistic Expectations:** Neuropathy is often a multifaceted condition with deep roots. It's unrealistic to expect a single product, treatment, or home remedy to provide a complete and lasting cure, especially in a short period.

- **Symptom Management Over Root Cause Resolution:** Many quick fixes focus solely on masking the symptoms of neuropathy, such as numbing creams or pain-relieving medications. While these can provide temporary relief, they don't address the underlying cause of the problem, leaving you stuck in a cycle of dependence and potentially allowing the condition to worsen over time.

- **Potential Risks and Side Effects:** As we discussed with supplements, even seemingly natural remedies can have unintended consequences, including adverse reactions, drug interactions, and unforeseen long-term effects.

- **The Placebo Effect: A Temporary Illusion:** The placebo effect—where our beliefs and expectations can influence our experience—is a powerful phenomenon. While a positive mindset can be beneficial for healing, the perceived benefits of a quick fix might stem from the placebo effect rather than any real therapeutic action. This can create a false sense of security, leading you to believe the underlying condition is improving when it's not.

Chasing after quick fixes can be a frustrating and expensive endeavor, leaving you feeling disillusioned and no closer to lasting relief. It's crucial to remember that true healing takes time, effort, and a commitment to addressing the root causes of your neuropathy.

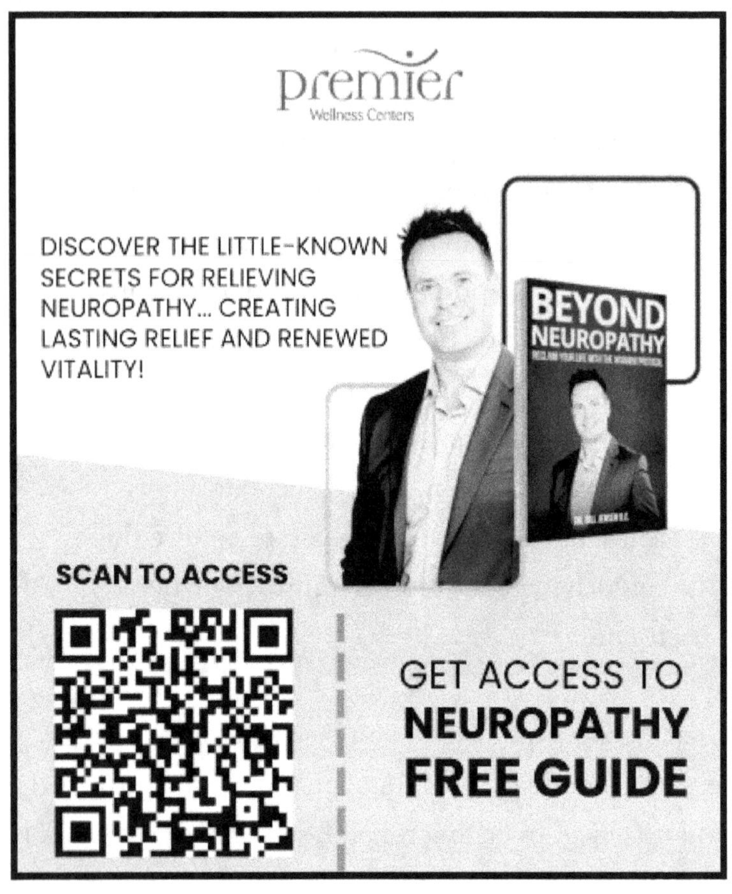

The Placebo Effect: When Belief Outweighs Reality

Our minds, like skilled artists, are constantly painting the landscapes of our reality. Sometimes, this inner canvas is flooded with pain and discomfort. The placebo effect offers us a powerful brushstroke—an opportunity to rewrite our own story.

Imagine yourself, gripping a pill, knowing deep down that it holds the power to alleviate your suffering. As you swallow it, a surge of hope and anticipation flows through your body. This is the essence of the placebo effect—an undeniable testament to the incredible capacity of the human mind to shape our own experiences.

However, it can sometimes muddy the waters of finding relief for neuropathy. Imagine yourself, desperate for a cure, stumbling across a promising new treatment online. All the testimonials rave about its success, and promises of a quick fix fill your mind with hope. You decide to give it a shot. Days or weeks later, you notice your symptoms easing. A surge of joy washes over you. Could this finally be the answer you've been searching for?

It's crucial to pause and consider the possibility that your newfound optimism is playing a part. The placebo effect, powerful and deceptive, might be leading you to believe a treatment is effective, even if its true efficacy is questionable. Just like a sugar pill, our minds can convince us of positive outcomes, even without a tangible change.

This is why it's vital to look beyond anecdotal evidence and testimonials when evaluating neuropathy treatments. Instead, prioritize evidence-based approaches:

- **Scientific Research:** Look for treatments backed by rigorous scientific studies published in reputable medical journals.
- **Clinical Trials:** Investigate whether the treatment has been tested in controlled clinical trials with statistically significant results.
- **Healthcare Professional Guidance:** Always consult with your healthcare provider to discuss any new treatment you're considering, especially if it lacks scientific backing or makes unrealistic promises.

Don't let the allure of a quick fix cloud your judgment. While hope is essential, it's crucial to temper that hope with a healthy dose of skepticism and a commitment to seeking out evidence-based solutions for lasting neuropathy relief.

Shifting the Focus: Embracing a Sustainable Path to Neuropathy Relief

In today's world, we're conditioned to expect instant results. However, neuropathy demands a different approach: a holistic focus on healing. It's not a simple

Band-Aid solution. Instead, think of it like nurturing a garden. It takes time, dedication, and an understanding of how interconnected factors affect your health. You're investing in the long-term, not just patching up symptoms.

Here's why embracing sustainable approaches is crucial for long-term neuropathy relief:

Early Diagnosis and Intervention:

Like many health conditions, early detection of neuropathy is paramount. The sooner you identify and address nerve damage, the better your chances of preventing further progression and improving your long-term outcome.

- **Don't Ignore the Early Signs:** If you're experiencing persistent tingling, numbness, pain, or weakness, don't dismiss it as "just getting older" or something you have to live with. Consult with your healthcare provider to determine the cause and explore treatment options.

- **Be Proactive with Underlying Conditions:** If you have a condition like diabetes that puts you at increased risk for neuropathy, work closely with your doctor to manage it effectively. This might involve medications, lifestyle modifications, or a combination of approaches.

Holistic Care for the Whole You:

Neuropathy is rarely caused by a single factor; it's often a complex interplay of genetic predisposition, lifestyle choices, environmental exposures, and underlying health conditions. Therefore, treating it effectively requires a holistic approach that addresses the whole person, not just the symptoms.

- **Personalized Treatment Plans:** Work with your healthcare provider to create a personalized treatment plan that considers your unique needs, medical history, and lifestyle. This might include a combination of conventional medical treatments, lifestyle modifications, complementary therapies, and nutritional counseling.
- **Address the Root Cause:** Don't settle for simply masking the symptoms. Focus on identifying and addressing the underlying causes of your neuropathy, whether it's blood sugar imbalances, nutritional deficiencies, autoimmune dysfunction, exposure to toxins, or other factors.

Embrace the Journey:

Healing from neuropathy is rarely a quick fix; it's an ongoing journey that requires patience, commitment, and a willingness to make sustainable lifestyle changes.

- **Celebrate Small Victories:** Don't get discouraged if you don't see results overnight. Focus on progress, not perfection. Celebrate each small victory along the way, whether it's a decrease in pain, improved balance, or simply a greater sense of hope.
- **Become an Empowered Patient:** Educate yourself about neuropathy, advocate for your needs, and actively participate in your healing journey.

By embracing a sustainable, holistic approach to neuropathy, you're not just treating a condition; you're investing in your long-term health and well-being.

Becoming Your Own Health Advocate: The Power of Patient Education

In the age of information overload, it's easy to feel overwhelmed, especially when you're facing a health challenge like neuropathy. It's tempting to grasp at straws, latching onto every promising headline or miracle cure advertised online. However, empowering yourself with accurate, evidence-based information is paramount for making informed decisions about your health and navigating the often-confusing world of neuropathy treatments.

Think of knowledge as your compass and informed decision-making as your map on the journey toward neuropathy relief.

Here's why patient education is so crucial:

- **Taking Control of Your Health:** When you understand your condition—its causes, symptoms, potential complications, and treatment options—you're empowered to make choices that align with your values and health goals.
- **Asking the Right Questions:** Knowledge enables you to engage in meaningful conversations with your healthcare providers. You'll be better equipped to ask informed questions, understand your treatment options, and advocate for your needs.
- **Discerning Fact from Fiction:** The internet is awash in misinformation about neuropathy treatments. By developing a discerning eye

for reliable sources and evidence-based practices, you can steer clear of misleading claims, potentially harmful remedies, and costly detours on your healing journey.

Seeking Reliable Sources of Information:

- **Consult Reputable Medical Organizations:** Turn to trusted sources such as:
    - Mayo Clinic
    - MedlinePlus
    - Department of Health and Human Services (HHS)
    - Centers for Disease Control and Prevention (CDC)
    - American Medical Association (AMA)
    - National Institutes of Health (NIH)
- **Connect with Patient Advocacy Groups:** Patient advocacy organizations often provide valuable information, resources, and support networks for those living with neuropathy.
- **Discuss Your Concerns with Your Doctor:** Your healthcare provider is your most trusted source for personalized medical advice and guidance.

Partnering with Healthcare Professionals:

Navigating neuropathy can be daunting, but at Premier Wellness Centers, your trusted chiropractic clinic, you don't have to face it alone. Our dedicated team provides comprehensive, evidence-based care, integrating the best of conventional medicine with holistic therapies to empower you on your journey toward relief. We're here to listen, answer your questions, and help you make informed decisions about your neuropathy care.

ACTION STEP: Scan the code below to download our 25 Anti-Inflammatory Recipes Guide.

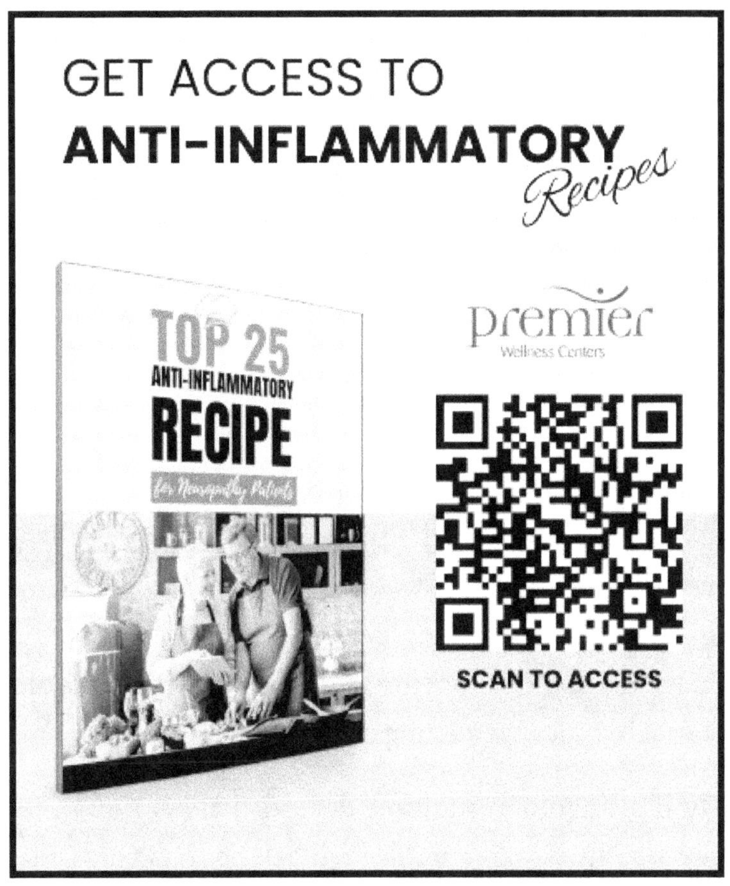

Unlock Your Path to Neuropathy Relief Now: Dial (772) 279-4145 to Speak With a Skilled Neuropathy Professional Today!

Individual results may vary. Please review the disclaimer after the Table of Contents.

7

———

DON'T LET NEUROPATHY DEFINE YOU: EMBRACE THESE TRUTHS AND RECLAIM YOUR LIFE

When I first met Susan, she was resigned to the belief that neuropathy would be a constant companion for the rest of her life. Years of living with numbness, tingling, and pain in her feet had convinced her that there was no hope for true relief, only the prospect of managing ever-worsening symptoms.

She'd been told by multiple doctors that her neuropathy was "incurable," a label that had chipped away at her spirit and left her feeling defeated. But when she came to PWC, a glimmer of hope flickered in her eyes—a hope that maybe, just maybe, there was a different path.

Susan embraced WARRIOR with a mix of cautious optimism and unwavering determination. She diligently followed her personalized treatment plan, attending therapy sessions, making dietary changes, incorporating gentle exercise into her routine, and even exploring stress-reducing practices like yoga and meditation.

The transformation was gradual but undeniable. The numbness in her feet began to recede, replaced by a tingling sensation that, while unusual at first, signaled a reawakening of her nerves. The pain lessened, her balance improved, and a newfound sense of vitality returned to her step.

Susan's journey is a powerful reminder that the label "incurable" doesn't have to be a life sentence. It's important to acknowledge that not everyone will experience the same benefits. However, her story highlights the potential for healing and the transformative power of a holistic approach that addresses the root causes of neuropathy, empowers the body's natural healing abilities, and reignites hope.

Challenging the "Incurable" Label

For far too long, the perception of neuropathy has been rooted in an assumption of incvitability, a bleak future marked by constant discomfort. While it's true that the condition presents complex challenges, dismissing it as simply an unchangeable fate does a disservice to both the patient and the evolving understanding of this neurological disorder. Research continues to provide insights and develop potential treatment avenues, giving us hope for a future where neuropathy isn't synonymous with a life confined by pain and limitations.

One of the most pervasive myths surrounding neuropathy is that it's always a one-way street, a progressive condition with no hope of a cure. This couldn't be further from the truth! While it's true that nerve damage can be challenging to relieve, it's not impossible. The truth is:

- **Neuropathy is not always progressive:** While some forms of neuropathy can worsen over time, many cases can be stabilized, prevented from progressing, or even significantly improved with the right interventions.
- **Early intervention is key:** Just like a fire is easier to extinguish when it's small, addressing neuropathy in its early stages, before significant nerve damage occurs, offers the best chance for successful treatment and symptom relief.

- **The underlying cause matters:** The possibility of symptom relief largely depends on the underlying cause of your neuropathy. If the cause is addressed effectively—whether it's controlling blood sugar, correcting a nutritional deficiency, treating an autoimmune condition, or reducing exposure to a toxin—nerve function can often be restored or significantly improved.

The WARRIOR Protocol, as we've discussed, is specifically designed to address the root causes of neuropathy and empower your body's natural healing abilities. By combining targeted therapies, lifestyle modifications, and nutritional support, we aim to not just manage symptoms but to create an internal environment where your nerves can regenerate and thrive.

While every case is unique, and we can never guarantee a "cure," we've witnessed remarkable transformations in our patients who've embraced this holistic approach. Don't let the "incurable" label define your journey. Hope, coupled with proactive action, can pave the way for lasting relief and a brighter future.

Pain is Not Your Partner: Why Ignoring Signals Delays Healing

We've often been taught to "tough it out" when it comes to pain, to push through discomfort and view it as a sign of weakness. However, this stoic approach can backfire, especially when it comes to chronic conditions like neuropathy. Enduring pain, especially when it's severe or persistent, doesn't build character; it can hinder healing and lead to more serious complications.

Our bodies are incredibly intelligent. Pain is a vital alarm system, a way for our body to communicate that something is wrong. It's a signal to pay attention, investigate, and take appropriate action. When we ignore these signals, we're essentially silencing a crucial communication channel, preventing our body from receiving the support it needs to heal.

Here are some potential negative consequences of ignoring pain signals:

- **Worsening Nerve Damage:** Pain often indicates ongoing nerve irritation or damage. Ignoring these signals allows the damage to progress, potentially leading to more severe symptoms, including loss of sensation, muscle weakness, and even permanent nerve dysfunction.

- **Increased Risk of Injury:** Neuropathy often affects balance and coordination, and numbness can mask injuries. Ignoring pain signals might lead you to push yourself beyond your limits, increasing your risk of falls, cuts, burns, or other injuries that you might not even realize you've sustained.

- **Chronic Pain and Reduced Quality of Life:** When pain persists unaddressed, it can lead to a downward spiral of chronic pain, sleep disturbances, emotional distress, and decreased quality of life.

Taking Action for Timely Recovery:

Early intervention is paramount. If you're experiencing persistent pain, numbness, tingling, or other neuropathy symptoms, don't wait for them to worsen. Seeking prompt medical attention can make a significant difference in your long-term outcome.

Here are the steps to take charge of your neuropathy journey:

1. **Early Intervention:** Don't ignore those early

warning signs. The sooner you seek help, the better.

2. **Data-Driven Analysis:** Premier Wellness Centers, a chiropractic clinic dedicated to your well-being, offers comprehensive neurological evaluations to assess nerve function, determine the underlying cause of your neuropathy, and develop a customized treatment plan to address your specific condition.

3. **Understanding Your Neuropathy:** Our experienced team provides comprehensive care focused on addressing the complexities of this condition. We'll take the time to listen to your concerns, answer your questions, and provide you with the support you need to make informed decisions about your health. This consultation is for informational purposes only and does not guarantee specific results. Every individual's condition and response to treatment varies.

Remember, you are your own best advocate. By listening to your body, seeking timely professional guidance, and embracing a proactive approach to your health, you can navigate the challenges of neuropathy with greater confidence and create a brighter, pain-free future.

Why a Comprehensive Approach Outweighs Quick Fixes

I know it can be frustrating – we all crave that simple solution, that magical cure that whisks away our pain. But, believe me, neuropathy is not a quick fix. It's like navigating a maze, with many paths that may lead nowhere. Focusing on a "miracle cure" can be incredibly disheartening, and worse, it can sometimes even do more harm than good.

Here's why the "miracle cure" for neuropathy is often a mirage:

- **Oversimplification of a Complex Condition:** Neuropathy is rarely a one-size-fits-all condition. It can stem from a wide range of causes, from blood sugar imbalances to autoimmune disorders to exposure to toxins. Attributing it to a single factor and attempting to address it with a single solution is like trying to solve a jigsaw puzzle with only one piece.
- **Medications: Masking Symptoms vs. Addressing Root Causes:** While medications

can play a role in managing neuropathy symptoms, they rarely address the underlying cause. Moreover, they often come with a long list of potential side effects that can range from mild to debilitating.

- **The Importance of Individualized Care:** Your body is unique, and your neuropathy treatment should reflect that. What works for one person might be ineffective or even detrimental for another. This highlights the crucial need for personalized care plans that consider your individual needs, medical history, lifestyle, and health goals.

Charting a Course for Sustainable Healing:

Instead of seeking a quick fix, consider these steps for a more comprehensive and ultimately more effective approach:

1. **Acknowledge the Complexity:** Recognize that neuropathy is often a multifaceted condition with various contributing factors. This understanding paves the way for a more holistic and effective treatment approach.
2. **Seek Professional Guidance:** Partner with a healthcare professional experienced in neuropathy care. They can help you identify

the root causes of your condition, assess the extent of nerve damage, and develop a personalized treatment plan.

3. **Embrace an Integrated Approach:** Integrative care combines the best of conventional medicine with evidence-informed complementary therapies to address all aspects of your well-being. This might include chiropractic care, physical therapy, nutritional counseling, stress management techniques, and lifestyle modifications tailored to your needs.

4. **Be Open to Innovation:** The field of neuropathy research is constantly evolving. Be open to exploring emerging therapies and technologies that align with your values and health goals.

True healing takes time, effort, and a commitment to addressing the root causes of your condition. By embracing a comprehensive, personalized, and holistic approach, you can move beyond the mirage of a miracle cure and embark on a path toward lasting relief, improved nerve health, and a more vibrant, fulfilling life.

Debunking the "Diabetes Only" Neuropathy Myth

It's true that diabetes is a major risk factor for neuropathy, often leading to a specific type known as diabetic neuropathy. However, this association has led to a common misconception: that neuropathy is exclusively linked to diabetes. This couldn't be further from the truth!

Neuropathy is like a malfunctioning alarm system; it can be triggered by a variety of culprits, not just high blood sugar. Imagine a house with a smoke alarm that can be set off by a fire in the kitchen, a faulty electrical wire, or even steam from a hot shower. Similarly, neuropathy can arise from a diverse range of causes:

- **Autoimmune Attacks:** In some cases, your own immune system, designed to protect you, can mistakenly attack your nerves as if they were foreign invaders. This occurs in conditions like Guillain-Barré syndrome, chronic inflammatory demyelinating polyneuropathy (CIDP), and lupus.
- **Infectious Invaders:** Certain infections, like Lyme disease, shingles, and HIV, can trigger an inflammatory response that damages nerves, leading to neuropathy.

- **Unseen Injuries:** Trauma to nerves, whether from car accidents, falls, sports injuries, or surgery, can disrupt nerve function and cause lasting pain and dysfunction.
- **Nutritional Deficiencies:** Your nerves rely on a steady supply of essential nutrients, particularly B vitamins. Deficiencies in these vitamins, often due to malabsorption or inadequate dietary intake, can lead to nerve damage and neuropathy.
- **Toxic Exposures:** Exposure to certain toxins, like heavy metals, pesticides, and some medications, can also damage nerves.
- **Inherited Conditions:** Some types of neuropathy are inherited, passed down through families due to genetic mutations.

This diverse range of causes underscores a crucial point: if you're experiencing neuropathy symptoms, don't assume it's solely due to diabetes, even if you have the condition. It's vital to seek a comprehensive evaluation to identify the root cause of your neuropathy, as this will guide your treatment plan and improve your chances of successful recovery.

Early recognition and intervention are crucial, regardless of the underlying cause. Don't ignore those persistent symptoms. By seeking prompt medical attention, you can address the problem at its source, prevent further nerve damage, and embark on a path toward lasting relief and improved well-being.

More Than Just Tingling: Recognizing Neuropathy's Hidden Signals

When we think of neuropathy, the first symptoms that often come to mind are tingling and numbness, especially in the hands and feet. While these are indeed common signs of nerve damage, it's important to recognize that neuropathy can manifest in a surprising variety of ways, often affecting seemingly unrelated parts of the body.

Think of your nervous system as a vast communication network, with nerves extending to every corner of your being. When these nerves are damaged, the consequences can reach far beyond those classic tingling sensations. Here are some lesser-known symptoms that often fly under the radar:

- **Unexplained Muscle Weakness:** You might find it harder to grip objects, button your shirt, climb stairs, or even stand for extended periods. This weakness can be a sign that neuropathy is affecting the nerves that control your muscles.

- **Stumbling and Fumbling: Balance Problems and Coordination Issues:** You might feel unsteady on your feet, prone to stumbling or tripping. You might also experience difficulty with fine motor skills, making it harder to button clothes, write, or handle small objects. This often stems from neuropathy affecting the nerves responsible for proprioception—your body's awareness of its position in space.

- **Digestive Distress:** Neuropathy can disrupt the nerves that control your digestive system, leading to a range of uncomfortable symptoms:
  - **Nausea and Vomiting:** You might experience unexplained bouts of nausea or vomiting, especially after meals.
  - **Constipation or Diarrhea:** Neuropathy can affect the muscles and nerves that control bowel movements, leading to either constipation or diarrhea.
  - **Gastroparesis:** In some cases, neuropathy can slow down stomach emptying, causing bloating, nausea, and a feeling of fullness after eating even small amounts.

- **Bladder and Bowel Troubles:** Neuropathy can also interfere with bladder and bowel function, leading to:
  - **Urinary Incontinence:** You might experience difficulty controlling your bladder, leading to leakage or urgency.
  - **Urinary Retention:** Conversely, some individuals with neuropathy find it difficult to fully empty their bladder.
  - **Bowel Incontinence:** Neuropathy can affect bowel control, leading to accidental leakage.
- **Intimacy Interrupted: Sexual Dysfunction:** Neuropathy can interfere with sexual function in both men and women, leading to:
  - **Erectile Dysfunction:** Men might experience difficulty achieving or maintaining an erection.
  - **Vaginal Dryness:** Women might experience reduced vaginal lubrication, making intercourse uncomfortable.
  - **Difficulty Achieving Orgasm:** Both men and women might find it challenging to reach orgasm.
- **Sweating Imbalances:** You might notice changes in your sweating patterns. Some individuals with neuropathy experience

excessive sweating, even when at rest, while others might find themselves sweating less than usual, even when they're hot.

- **Heightened Sensitivity:** Neuropathy can make your skin more sensitive to touch, temperature, or even clothing. What might normally feel like a gentle touch could feel painful or uncomfortable.

It's crucial to remember that neuropathy can present a wide range of symptoms beyond the typical tingling and numbness. Recognizing these lesser-known signs is vital for early diagnosis and treatment. If you're experiencing any unusual or persistent symptoms, don't dismiss them. Consult with your healthcare provider to determine the cause and explore treatment options. The sooner you address nerve damage, the better your chances of preventing further progression and reclaiming your health and well-being.

This chapter has illuminated the importance of challenging common misconceptions surrounding neuropathy. By dispelling these myths and understanding the full spectrum of symptoms, we can empower ourselves to seek timely intervention, explore effective treatment options, and embrace a hopeful outlook. Remember, neuropathy doesn't have to define your life. With knowledge, proactive action, and the support of experienced healthcare professionals, you can navigate the challenges, reclaim your health, and live a full and vibrant life.

ACTION STEP: Take our free Nerve Damage Evaluation by scanning this code:

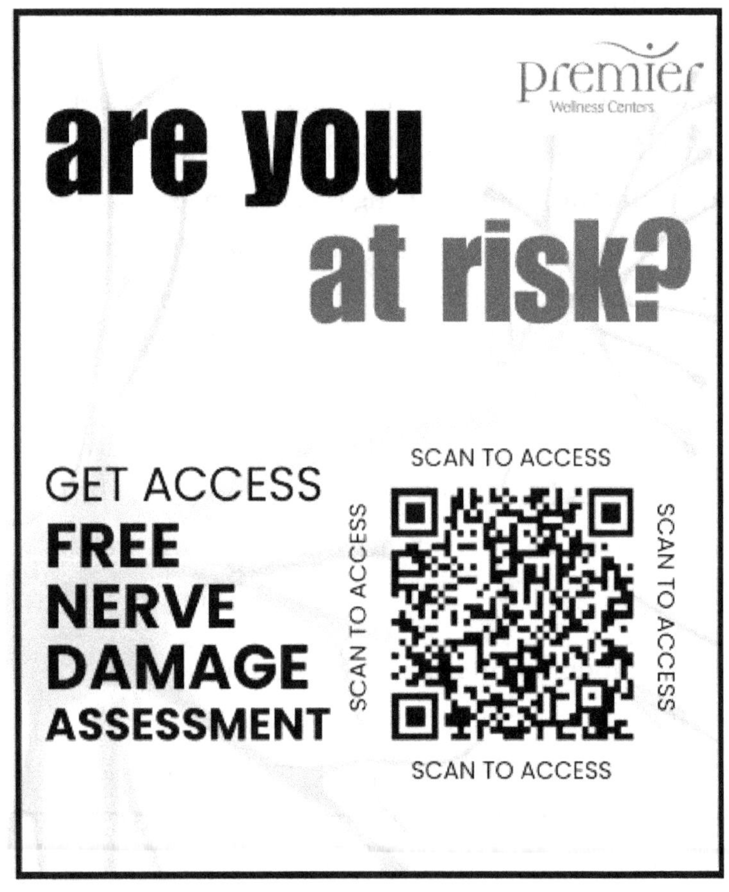

Unlock Your Path to Neuropathy Relief Now: Dial (772) 279-4145 to Speak With a Skilled Neuropathy Professional Today!

Individual results may vary. Please review the disclaimer after the Table of Contents.

8

NERVES ON HIGH ALERT: UNDERSTANDING YOUR BODY'S COMMAND CENTER

I remember the day Michael walked into my office, his face etched with worry. A recent diagnosis of peripheral neuropathy had left him feeling like his body had betrayed him. The numbness in his hands made it difficult to button his shirt or grip a pen, and the tingling in his feet made walking feel like navigating a minefield of pins and needles. He felt disconnected from his own body, the once-familiar sensations replaced by a disconcerting silence.

As we discussed his condition, I explained the intricate workings of the nervous system—that remarkable communication network that orchestrates every sensation, movement, and function within our bodies. I described how neuropathy disrupts this intricate network, like creating roadblocks or static on the communication lines, leading to those frustrating and often-frightening symptoms.

Michael was a visual learner, so I used diagrams and analogies to help him understand how WARRIOR could address the root causes of his neuropathy, promote nerve regeneration, and restore the flow of communication throughout his body.

He embraced the program with a dedication that inspired me, diligently attending his therapy sessions, making dietary changes, and incorporating gentle exercise into his routine. Over time, the numbness gradually subsided, the tingling lessened, and a sense of reconnection returned to his body. He regained dexterity in his hands, his gait became more steady, and the fear in his eyes was replaced by a glimmer of hope.

It's important to note that every individual's experience with neuropathy and their response to treatment is unique. However, Michael's journey highlights a crucial point: understanding the complexities of our nervous system empowers us to approach healing with greater clarity and purpose.

Your Body's Information Superhighway: A Closer Look at the Nervous System

Our bodies are truly marvels of engineering. Trillions of cells constantly chatter amongst themselves, like tiny voices whispering in the grand, bustling marketplace that is your body. This remarkable community thrives because of a magnificent network of nerves, the nervous system, acting like a superhighway for information flow. From controlling your heartbeat and breathing, to helping you learn, create, and feel, this intricate network is the heart of your body's communication, constantly buzzing with activity.

This vast communication network is divided into two main branches:

1. The Central Nervous System (CNS): The Control Tower

The CNS, consisting of your brain and spinal cord, is like the city's central control tower, receiving information from all parts of your body, processing it, and sending out instructions.

- **The Brain: The Mastermind:** Your brain is the ultimate control center, responsible for your thoughts, emotions, memories, movements, and every sensation you experience.

- **The Spinal Cord: The Information Conduit:** Your spinal cord acts as the primary communication pathway between your brain and the rest of your body. It's like a superhighway, transmitting messages to and from the brain, enabling you to move, feel, and respond to your environment.

2. The Peripheral Nervous System (PNS): The Network of Messengers

The PNS consists of all the nerves that extend from your brain and spinal cord, reaching out to every corner of your body. These nerves act like tireless messengers, carrying information to and from the CNS, allowing you to interact with your surroundings and control your bodily functions.

The PNS is further divided into two branches:

- **The Somatic Nervous System: Controlling Voluntary Movements:** This branch controls your voluntary movements—the actions you consciously choose to perform, like walking, talking, and waving your hand.

- **The Autonomic Nervous System: Managing Automatic Functions:** This branch operates behind the scenes, regulating vital functions that you don't consciously control, like your heartbeat, breathing, digestion, and blood pressure.

Understanding these two branches of your nervous system is crucial for comprehending how neuropathy disrupts this intricate communication network. When nerves in the PNS are damaged, it's like creating roadblocks or cutting communication lines in that bustling city, leading to a range of symptoms and dysfunction.

Anatomy of a Nerve: Understanding How Neuropathy Disrupts the Lines of Communication

Imagine a neuron as a long, slender wire, carefully insulated to transmit electrical signals efficiently. That's essentially how your nerves function. They're designed to carry messages throughout your body, enabling you to feel sensations, control your muscles, and regulate your bodily functions.

Here's a closer look at the structure of a typical nerve:

- **The Axon: The Signal Conductor:** The axon is the long, slender projection of a neuron that carries electrical impulses away from the cell body, like a wire transmitting electricity.

- **Myelin Sheath: The Protective Insulation:** Many axons are wrapped in a fatty substance called myelin, which acts like insulation around an electrical wire, speeding up the transmission of nerve impulses and preventing signal leakage.
- **Nerve Endings: The Signal Transmitters:** At the end of the axon are nerve endings, which release chemical messengers called neurotransmitters to communicate with other neurons, muscles, or glands.

Now, let's explore how neuropathy disrupts this intricate structure:

- **Damage to the Axon:** When the axon is damaged, it can disrupt or block the transmission of nerve impulses, like a frayed wire that can't carry electricity effectively. This can lead to weakness, numbness, and loss of sensation.
- **Myelin Breakdown:** In some types of neuropathy, the myelin sheath is damaged or destroyed. This is like stripping the

insulation off an electrical wire, causing signal leakage, slowed transmission, and interference with nerve communication. This can lead to a range of symptoms, including tingling, burning pain, muscle weakness, and coordination problems.

- **Impaired Neurotransmitter Release:** Neuropathy can also affect the nerve endings, impairing their ability to release neurotransmitters effectively. This disruption in chemical communication can lead to a variety of symptoms, depending on the type of nerve affected.

Our nervous system is a marvel of intricate pathways, carrying messages between our brain and every part of our body. Imagine these pathways being disrupted, the flow of information hindered, and the signals becoming scrambled. That's the reality of neuropathy. It's like a power outage in the central command system, causing malfunctions throughout. From the tingling sensation in your limbs to potential weakness in your muscles, loss of balance, and even issues with internal organ function, neuropathy can significantly impact our quality of life.

The Many Faces of Neuropathy: Understanding the Different Types

Neuropathy is not a single condition but rather an umbrella term encompassing a wide range of disorders that affect the peripheral nerves—those nerves that extend beyond your brain and spinal cord. Just as there are different types of roads in that bustling city—highways, side streets, and back alleys—there are various forms of neuropathy, each with its unique characteristics, causes, and symptoms.

Here are some of the most common types of neuropathy:

- **Diabetic Neuropathy:** As the name suggests, this type of neuropathy is a common complication of diabetes, both type 1 and type 2. Chronically elevated blood sugar damages the delicate blood vessels that nourish your nerves, leading to a range of symptoms, most often starting in the feet and legs.
- **Peripheral Neuropathy:** This is a general term referring to neuropathy that affects the nerves in the extremities—your hands, feet, arms, and legs. It can be caused by a variety

of factors, including diabetes, alcoholism, vitamin deficiencies, autoimmune diseases, and exposure to toxins.

- **Autonomic Neuropathy:** This type affects the nerves that control your involuntary bodily functions—your heart rate, blood pressure, digestion, bladder control, and sexual function. It often occurs in conjunction with other types of neuropathy, particularly diabetic neuropathy.
- **Focal Neuropathy:** This type affects a single nerve or a group of nerves, often causing sudden weakness or pain in a specific area, such as the wrist (carpal tunnel syndrome), the face (Bell's palsy), or the thigh (meralgia paresthetica).
- **Proximal Neuropathy:** This type, also known as diabetic amyotrophy, primarily affects the nerves in the hips, thighs, and buttocks, causing pain, weakness, and muscle wasting. It's more common in people with type 2 diabetes.
- **Sensory Neuropathy:** This type primarily affects the nerves that carry sensory information, like touch, temperature, and pain, leading to numbness, tingling, burning sensations, and heightened sensitivity.

- **Motor Neuropathy:** This type primarily affects the nerves that control muscle movement, leading to weakness, cramps, muscle twitching, and difficulty with coordination and balance.
- **Small Fiber Neuropathy:** This type affects the small nerve fibers responsible for transmitting pain and temperature sensations. It often causes burning pain, especially in the feet, and can also affect autonomic functions like sweating and heart rate.

Understanding the different types of neuropathy can help you and your healthcare provider determine the most appropriate course of treatment and develop a personalized plan to address your specific needs.

Unmasking the Culprits: Unearthing the Root Causes of Neuropathy

Neuropathy is rarely a simple condition with a single, easily identifiable cause. It's often the result of a complex interplay of factors that can damage or disrupt the delicate communication network of your peripheral nerves. Think of it like a mystery novel, where you need to gather clues and piece together the evidence to uncover the true culprit.

Here are some of the most common culprits behind neuropathy:

- **Blood Sugar Imbalances:** Chronically elevated blood sugar, a hallmark of diabetes, is a leading cause of neuropathy. High blood sugar damages the tiny blood vessels that supply your nerves with oxygen and nutrients, leading to nerve dysfunction and degeneration.
- **Inflammatory Fires:** Inflammation, your body's natural response to injury or infection, can become a destructive force when it's chronic and uncontrolled. This relentless inflammation can damage nerve cells, disrupt nerve signaling, and contribute to pain and other neuropathy symptoms.
- **Nutritional Deficiencies:** Your nerves rely on a steady supply of essential vitamins, minerals, and antioxidants to function optimally. Deficiencies in B vitamins, particularly B12, B6, and folate, are common culprits behind neuropathy.
- **Underlying Medical Conditions:** A wide range of medical conditions can contribute to neuropathy, including:

- ○ **Autoimmune Diseases:** In conditions like lupus, rheumatoid arthritis, and Guillain-Barré syndrome, your immune system mistakenly attacks your own tissues, including your nerves.
  - ○ **Kidney Disease:** Kidney dysfunction can lead to a buildup of toxins in the blood that can damage nerves.
  - ○ **Hypothyroidism:** An underactive thyroid gland can slow down metabolism and contribute to nerve damage.
- **Exposure to Toxins:** Exposure to certain toxins, like heavy metals, pesticides, industrial solvents, and some medications, can damage nerves and lead to neuropathy.
- **Physical Injuries:** Trauma to nerves, whether from car accidents, falls, sports injuries, or surgery, can disrupt nerve function and cause lasting pain and dysfunction.
- **Genetic Predisposition:** In some cases, neuropathy runs in families, indicating a genetic predisposition to nerve damage.

Why Addressing Root Causes is Paramount:

Imagine a dripping faucet, constantly creating a puddle on your floor. Wiping it up provides temporary relief but doesn't fix the problem.

Similarly, pain medications for neuropathy might mask the symptoms, but they won't address the underlying issue.

Neuropathy, at its core, is a disruption of nerve function. Addressing the root cause, whether it be diabetes, vitamin deficiency, or other factors, allows your body to heal and restore nerve health. It's about empowering your body to repair itself, offering long-term relief and improving quality of life.

Awaken Your Inner Healer: Tapping into the Power of Neuroplasticity

For years, the prevailing belief in neuroscience was that the adult brain was relatively fixed—that once nerve cells were damaged, they couldn't regenerate. However, groundbreaking research in recent decades has revealed a remarkable truth: our brains and nervous systems possess an extraordinary capacity for change and adaptation, a phenomenon known as neuroplasticity.

Think of your brain as a dynamic, ever-evolving landscape, constantly rewiring and reorganizing itself in response to experiences, learning, and even injury. This remarkable ability means that even when nerves are damaged, they have the potential to heal, regenerate, and form new connections.

While the extent of nerve regeneration can vary depending on the severity and type of neuropathy, there are steps you can take to support your body's natural healing processes:

1. Fueling Nerve Regeneration: The Power of Targeted Nutrition

Remember, your nerves require a steady supply of specific nutrients to function optimally and repair damage.

- **B Vitamins: The Nerve Essentials:** B vitamins, particularly B12, B6, and folate, are crucial for nerve cell growth, repair, and the production of neurotransmitters—those chemical messengers that enable nerve communication.
- **Antioxidants: The Damage Defenders:** Antioxidants like vitamins C and E, alpha-lipoic acid, and glutathione help protect nerve cells from damage caused by free radicals.
- **Omega-3 Fatty Acids: The Building Blocks:** These essential fats are vital components of

nerve cell membranes, supporting their structure and function.

2. Creating a Healing Environment: Lifestyle Adjustments That Matter

- **Blood Sugar Control:** If you have diabetes, maintaining stable blood sugar levels is paramount for preventing further nerve damage and supporting nerve healing.
- **Regular Exercise:** As we've discussed, exercise enhances blood flow to your nerves, delivers vital nutrients, and stimulates nerve regeneration.
- **Stress Management:** Chronic stress can exacerbate neuropathy symptoms and hinder healing. Incorporating stress-reducing techniques like mindfulness, meditation, yoga, or deep breathing exercises can promote a more healing internal environment.

3. The WARRIOR Protocol: A Holistic Approach to Nerve Regeneration

WARRIOR, as you've learned, is designed to address the root causes of neuropathy and support your body's natural healing abilities through a comprehensive combination of:

W – Water Hydration: Optimizing hydration is essential for flushing toxins, improving circulation, and supporting overall nerve function.

A – Anti-Inflammatory: Reducing chronic inflammation throughout the body is crucial for protecting nerves from damage and creating an environment where they can heal.

R – Revitalize Blood Flow: Enhancing blood flow delivers vital oxygen and nutrients to damaged nerves, promoting their regeneration and restoration.

R – Restoration of Tissue Health: Supporting the body's natural healing processes is essential for repairing damaged nerve tissues and restoring their structural integrity.

I – Improve Oxygenation: Increasing oxygen delivery to nerve cells is crucial for enhancing their function and accelerating the healing process.

O – Optimize Nutrition: Providing your body with the right nutrients is essential for supporting nerve health, repair, and regeneration.

R – Rehabilitation & Functional Movement: Engaging in targeted exercises and therapies helps to strengthen muscles, improve balance and coordination, and enhance overall functional capacity.

The human brain has an incredible ability to adapt and heal, a process known as neuroplasticity. By utilizing targeted nutrition, modifying lifestyle habits, and incorporating the WARRIOR method, individuals can promote nerve regeneration and recovery. This holistic approach aims to facilitate the restoration of lost function, offering a path towards a fulfilling life.

Patience and Persistence: Why Time and Consistency Are Your Greatest Allies

Healing from neuropathy is rarely a sprint; it's more akin to a marathon. It's a journey that requires patience, persistence, and a deep understanding that your body's healing processes unfold in their own time.

Think of it this way: imagine planting a seed in the ground. You wouldn't expect it to sprout into a towering tree overnight, would you? It takes time, nourishment, and consistent care for that tiny seed to develop roots, send up a fragile shoot, and eventually grow into a strong, resilient tree.

Nerve healing follows a similar trajectory. When nerves are damaged, it takes time for them to repair, regenerate, and reestablish those crucial communication pathways. This healing process can't be rushed; it unfolds gradually, often in subtle increments that might not be immediately noticeable.

Here's why time and consistency are essential for neuropathy recovery:

- **Nerve Regeneration is a Gradual Process:** Nerves regenerate at a slow pace, often only about an inch per month. This means that significant healing can take weeks, months, or even years, depending on the severity of the damage and the individual's overall health.
- **Consistency Creates Momentum:** Just as a single workout won't transform your fitness overnight, sporadic efforts at managing neuropathy won't yield lasting results. Consistency is key. Whether it's adhering to your treatment plan, making dietary changes, incorporating daily exercise, or managing stress, consistent effort over time creates momentum for healing.
- **Building New Habits Takes Time:** Lifestyle modifications, such as adopting a healthy

diet or establishing a regular exercise routine, require patience and persistence. Don't get discouraged if you slip up or have setbacks along the way. Gently guide yourself back to your healthy habits, knowing that each small step contributes to the larger goal of healing.

- **Patience Fosters Resilience:** Healing from neuropathy can be a challenging journey. There might be days when you feel discouraged or frustrated. Cultivating patience allows you to weather these inevitable ups and downs, knowing that your consistent efforts are setting the stage for long-term healing and improved well-being.

Your body is a remarkable healing machine, but it needs time and consistent support to do its job effectively. By embracing patience as a virtue and persistence as a guiding principle, you can create a fertile ground for nerve regeneration, reclaim lost function, and emerge from your neuropathy journey stronger and more resilient than ever before.

Our bodies are truly amazing, intricately woven together by a delicate network of nerves. But sometimes, this intricate system is thrown off balance, leaving us feeling like we're trapped in our own bodies due to neuropathy. But fear not! The human body is a remarkable architect, able to rebuild and restore even its most delicate components. Through a deeper understanding of the causes of neuropathy and by actively promoting nerve regeneration, we can find our way back to a life filled with vibrant health and renewed hope.

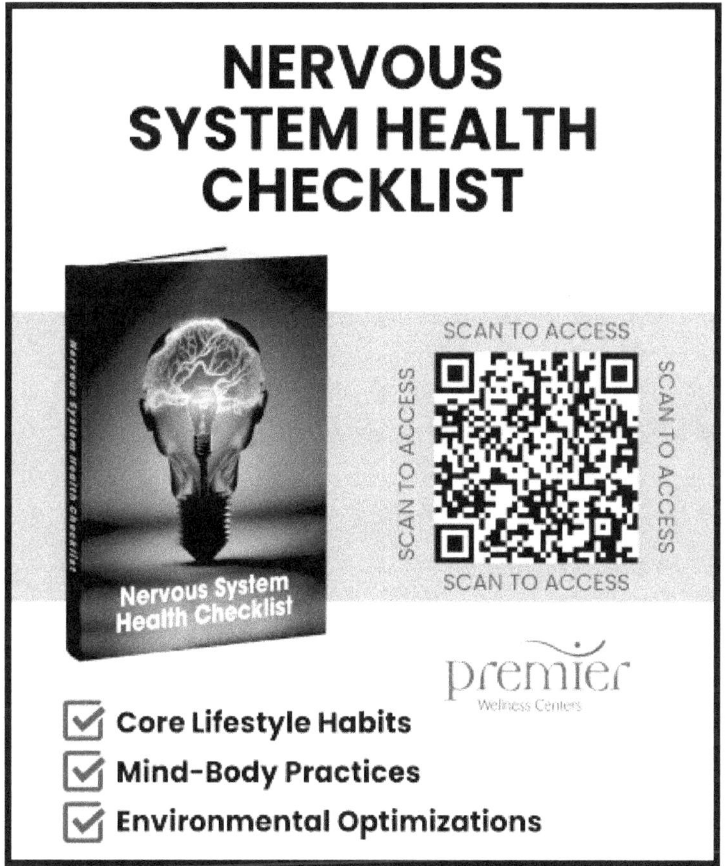

Unlock Your Path to Neuropathy Relief Now: Dial (772) 279-4145 to Speak With a Skilled Neuropathy Professional Today!

Individual results may vary. Please review the disclaimer after the Table of Contents.

9

———

STATINS AND YOUR NERVES: UNDERSTANDING THE POTENTIAL RISKS AND BENEFITS

I recall a patient, Emily, who came to me with a mix of relief and apprehension. She'd recently been prescribed statins to manage her high cholesterol, a decision she'd made after a heart-to-heart with her cardiologist. She understood the importance of protecting her heart, but a nagging worry lingered in her mind—the potential for statin-induced neuropathy.

Emily had a family history of neuropathy, and the thought of experiencing those debilitating symptoms —the numbness, the tingling, the pain—filled her with dread. We discussed her concerns, carefully weighing the potential benefits of statins for her heart health against the potential risks of nerve damage.

I explained that while statins are essential for many, they're not a one-size-fits-all solution, and there are ways to mitigate the risks. We incorporated the principles of the WARRIOR Protocol, focusing on enhancing her nutrition, supporting nerve health with targeted supplements like CoQ10, and addressing lifestyle factors that could contribute to inflammation and nerve damage.

Emily's proactive approach paid off. She diligently followed her personalized plan, and not only did her cholesterol levels improve, but she also managed to avoid the nerve-related side effects she'd feared. It's important to remember that individual responses to medications vary, and this is just one person's experience. However, Emily's story highlights a crucial point: we have more power than we often realize to influence our health outcomes, even when medications are necessary.

This brings us to a crucial conversation about statins —those little pills that have become both a blessing and a potential curse in the realm of heart health. They have become a lifeline for many battling high cholesterol, offering a powerful shield against heart attacks and strokes. They've been instrumental in saving countless lives, ushering in a new era of preventative care. However, as with any medication, there's a catch. Some individuals may experience nerve damage as a side effect, a painful complication known as neuropathy.

This delicate dance between heart protection and potential nerve damage creates a difficult decision for those at risk, especially those who already suffer from nerve-related conditions or those with diabetes, which makes them more susceptible to neuropathy.

Here's what's important to understand:

- **Statins' Cholesterol-Lowering Power:** Statins work by blocking an enzyme in the liver that produces cholesterol. By lowering cholesterol levels, particularly LDL cholesterol (often referred to as "bad" cholesterol), statins can reduce the buildup of plaque in arteries, lowering the risk of heart attacks, strokes, and other cardiovascular events.
- **The Neuropathy Connection:** While statins are generally safe for most people, some individuals experience muscle aches, weakness, and even neuropathy as a side effect. The exact mechanisms behind statin-induced neuropathy aren't fully understood, but some theories suggest that statins might

interfere with the production of CoQ10, a nutrient essential for nerve health.

- **Individualized Risk vs. Benefit:** The decision to take statins, and which type of statin to use, should always be made in consultation with your healthcare provider. They can assess your individual risk factors for heart disease, your current health status, and your potential risk of developing neuropathy to help you make an informed decision.

Lowering cholesterol isn't a one-size-fits-all situation. You've got options! There are plenty of ways to manage your cholesterol levels and keep your heart healthy. From simple lifestyle changes and dietary adjustments to different medications, it's about finding what works best for you. The goal is to keep your heart happy without putting your nerves at risk.

Statins Under the Microscope: Understanding Cholesterol Reduction and the CoQ10 Connection

To comprehend how statins might contribute to neuropathy, it's helpful to delve deeper into their mechanism of action—how they work on a cellular level.

- **Cholesterol Control:** Your liver is a cholesterol-producing powerhouse, manufacturing this waxy substance that's essential for various bodily functions, including cell membrane structure and hormone production. However, high levels of cholesterol, particularly LDL cholesterol, can lead to a buildup of plaque in your arteries, increasing your risk of heart disease. Statins step in to block an enzyme called HMG-CoA reductase, a key player in cholesterol production. By inhibiting this enzyme, statins effectively reduce the amount of cholesterol your liver produces, lowering your overall cholesterol levels.

- **The CoQ10 Conundrum:** While statins excel at lowering cholesterol, their interference with the HMG-CoA reductase enzyme has a ripple effect on another crucial pathway—the production of CoQ10 (coenzyme Q10). CoQ10 is a potent antioxidant that plays a vital role in cellular energy production, particularly within the mitochondria, the powerhouses of your cells. Your nerves, with their high energy demands, are particularly reliant on adequate CoQ10 levels for optimal function.

- **When CoQ10 Levels Dip:** When statins lower cholesterol, they also tend to lower CoQ10 levels, potentially creating an energy deficit within nerve cells. This disruption in energy production can impair nerve function, leading to those familiar neuropathy symptoms—tingling, numbness, pain, and weakness.

Think of it this way: Imagine your nerve cells as cars reliant on gasoline to function. CoQ10 is like the spark plug, essential for igniting the fuel and generating energy. Statins, while effectively lowering cholesterol (like removing excess oil), might inadvertently affect the spark plug (CoQ10), leading to engine troubles (nerve dysfunction).

It's important to note that not everyone who takes statins develops neuropathy. The risk varies depending on individual factors like genetics, dosage, duration of statin use, and the presence of other health conditions like diabetes. However, understanding this potential link between statins and CoQ10 depletion sheds light on why some individuals experience nerve-related side effects from these commonly prescribed medications.

CoQ10: The Nerve Protector Depleted by Statins

We've touched on the link between statins, CoQ10 depletion, and neuropathy, but let's delve deeper into why CoQ10 is so crucial for nerve health and explore the spectrum of potential side effects associated with statins.

CoQ10: Your Nerves' Energy Spark Plug

Think of CoQ10 as a tiny but mighty powerhouse within your cells, playing a vital role in energy production. Your nerves, with their constant demand for energy to transmit signals throughout your body, are particularly reliant on adequate CoQ10 levels.

This potent antioxidant also serves as a protector, shielding your nerve cells from damage caused by free radicals—those unstable molecules that can wreak havoc on cellular structures. Without sufficient CoQ10, your nerves become more vulnerable to oxidative stress, inflammation, and ultimately, dysfunction.

Beyond Neuropathy: Statins' Potential Side Effects

While statins are generally safe and effective for many people, it's essential to be aware of their potential side effects, which can range from mild to severe.

- **Muscle Aches and Weakness:** The most common side effect of statins is muscle aches and weakness (myalgia). This can range from mild discomfort to debilitating pain, making everyday activities challenging.

- **Liver Enzyme Elevation:** Statins can sometimes cause an elevation in liver enzymes, a sign of potential liver damage. Regular monitoring of liver function is essential for those taking statins.
- **Increased Blood Sugar:** Some studies have suggested that statins might slightly increase the risk of developing type 2 diabetes. This is particularly concerning for individuals already at risk for diabetes or those with prediabetes.
- **Cognitive Effects:** While less common, some individuals report cognitive side effects from statins, such as memory problems, confusion, or difficulty concentrating.
- **Other Rare Side Effects:** In rare cases, statins can cause more serious side effects, such as severe muscle damage (rhabdomyolysis), tendon problems, or allergic reactions.

It's crucial to have open and honest conversations with your healthcare provider about your medications, including statins. Discuss any side effects you're experiencing, as well as your concerns about potential risks.

Decoding the Data: Research Insights into Statins and Neuropathy

While the connection between statins and neuropathy is complex, research is shedding light on factors that might increase the risk of developing nerve-related side effects from these cholesterol-lowering medications.

Here are some key risk factors to consider:

- **Pre-Existing Neuropathy or Diabetes:** If you already have neuropathy or diabetes, you're at a higher risk of experiencing statin-induced neuropathy. This is because your nerves might already be compromised, making them more susceptible to further damage from CoQ10 depletion or other statin-related effects.
- **Advanced Age:** As we age, our bodies naturally produce less CoQ10, and our nerves become more vulnerable to damage. This makes older adults more susceptible to statin-induced neuropathy.

- **Polypharmacy (Taking Multiple Medications):** Taking multiple medications, especially those that can also affect nerve health or interfere with CoQ10 production, can increase your risk of neuropathy.
- **Vitamin D Deficiency:** Vitamin D plays a vital role in nerve health, and a deficiency in this crucial nutrient has been linked to an increased risk of neuropathy, including statin-induced neuropathy.
- **Genetic Predisposition:** Some individuals might have a genetic predisposition that makes them more sensitive to statin-related side effects, including neuropathy.
- **Dosage and Duration of Statin Use:** Higher doses of statins and longer durations of use have been associated with an increased risk of neuropathy.
- **Underlying Health Conditions:** Certain health conditions, such as hypothyroidism, kidney disease, and liver disease, can also increase your susceptibility to statin-induced neuropathy.

While these risk factors can help identify individuals who might be more vulnerable to statin-related neuropathy, it's important to remember that not everyone who has these risk factors will develop neuropathy. The decision to take statins should be made on a case-by-case basis, carefully weighing the potential benefits for heart health against the potential risks of side effects.

The Hidden Danger: Misdiagnosis and the Importance of Open Communication

One of the most concerning aspects of statin-induced neuropathy is the potential for misdiagnosis. Since neuropathy can stem from a variety of causes, its symptoms might be mistakenly attributed to other conditions, particularly in individuals with existing health issues like diabetes.

This misdiagnosis can have serious consequences:

- **Delayed Treatment:** If statin-induced neuropathy is misdiagnosed, appropriate treatment might be delayed, allowing nerve damage to progress further.
- **Unnecessary Treatments and Tests:** A misdiagnosis can lead to unnecessary treatments and tests, adding to healthcare costs and potentially causing additional side effects or complications.
- **Increased Risk of Complications:** Untreated neuropathy can lead to a range of

complications, including falls, injuries, infections, and a decreased quality of life.

Open Communication: Your Best Defense

The key to preventing misdiagnosis and ensuring appropriate care is open and honest communication with your healthcare provider.

- **Report Any New Symptoms:** If you're taking statins and start experiencing any new symptoms, especially tingling, numbness, pain, or weakness, don't hesitate to report them to your doctor.
- **Keep a Symptom Journal:** Keeping a journal of your symptoms, including when they started, how often they occur, and their severity, can be helpful for your doctor to assess the situation.
- **Discuss Your Concerns:** If you're concerned about the potential risks of statins, or if you're already experiencing neuropathy symptoms, don't be afraid to discuss your concerns with your doctor.
- **Explore Alternatives:** Remember, statins aren't the only option for managing cholesterol levels and reducing heart disease risk. Work with your doctor to explore

alternative approaches that might be more suitable for your individual needs and health history.

Your health is a partnership. By being an active participant in your care, communicating openly with your doctor, and staying informed about your medications, you can make the best decisions for your overall well-being.

Nurturing Heart Health Naturally

While statins have undoubtedly played a significant role in preventing heart disease, they're not the only path to cardiovascular well-being. In fact, focusing solely on lowering cholesterol with medication often overlooks the underlying causes of heart disease, which are often rooted in lifestyle and dietary factors.

Think of it this way: Imagine trying to fix a leaky roof by simply placing buckets underneath to catch the drips. You might temporarily contain the problem, but you're not addressing the source of the leak. Similarly, solely relying on medication to lower cholesterol without addressing lifestyle factors that contribute to heart disease is like constantly emptying those buckets without ever fixing the roof.

Let's shift the focus to addressing those root causes, nurturing heart health from the inside out:

Taming the Flames of Inflammation:

Chronic inflammation is like a smoldering fire within your body, silently damaging blood vessels and contributing to the development of plaque buildup— a hallmark of heart disease.

- **Embrace an Anti-Inflammatory Diet:** Load up on foods rich in antioxidants and omega-3 fatty acids, such as colorful fruits and vegetables, fatty fish, nuts, seeds, and olive oil. These foods help calm inflammation and protect your cardiovascular system.
- **Reduce Processed Foods:** Processed foods, laden with unhealthy fats, added sugars, and artificial ingredients, often fuel inflammation. Minimize your intake of these processed options and prioritize whole, unprocessed foods.
- **Manage Stress:** Chronic stress contributes to inflammation throughout the body. Embrace stress-reducing techniques like mindfulness, meditation, yoga, or spending time in nature.

Fighting Oxidative Stress:

Oxidative stress occurs when there's an imbalance between free radicals (unstable molecules that damage cells) and antioxidants (compounds that neutralize free radicals). This imbalance can damage blood vessels and contribute to heart disease.

- **Boost Your Antioxidant Intake:** Load up on colorful fruits and vegetables, which are packed with antioxidants.
- **Choose Healthy Fats:** Healthy fats, like those found in avocados, olive oil, nuts, and fatty fish, provide antioxidant protection.
- **Limit Exposure to Toxins:** Exposure to environmental toxins, like cigarette smoke, pollution, and pesticides, can increase oxidative stress.

Other Root Causes to Address:

- **Blood Sugar Imbalances:** High blood sugar, whether from diabetes or prediabetes, damages blood vessels and significantly increases the risk of heart disease.
- **Physical Inactivity:** A sedentary lifestyle contributes to a whole host of health problems, including heart disease.

- **Smoking:** Smoking is one of the most significant risk factors for heart disease.

By addressing these root causes through lifestyle modifications, a nutrient-rich diet, and stress management techniques, you can create a more heart-healthy environment from within, reducing your reliance on medications and promoting long-term well-being.

Statin Decisions: Your Health, Your Choice

Deciding whether to take statins, and which type of statin is right for you, is a personal choice that should be made in close consultation with your healthcare provider. It's a decision that requires careful consideration of your individual risk factors, potential benefits, and potential risks.

Here are some key points to guide your decision-making:

- **Open Communication is Paramount:** Discuss your concerns openly and honestly with your doctor. Share your medical history, any existing health conditions, medications you're currently taking, and any side effects you're experiencing.

- **Individualized Risk Assessment:** Work with your doctor to assess your individual risk factors for heart disease. This includes considering factors like family history, cholesterol levels, blood pressure, smoking history, age, and lifestyle.

- **Weighing Benefits and Risks:** Carefully weigh the potential benefits of statins in reducing your risk of heart attacks and strokes against the potential risks of side effects, including muscle aches, liver problems, blood sugar fluctuations, and neuropathy.

- **Exploring Alternatives:** Remember, statins aren't the only option for managing cholesterol and reducing heart disease risk. Discuss lifestyle modifications, dietary changes, and other medications with your doctor to find the approach that best suits your needs.

Here are some key questions to ask your doctor about statins:

- Based on my individual risk factors, what are the potential benefits of statins for me?

- What are the potential risks and side effects of statins, and how likely am I to experience them?
- Are there any specific types of statins that might be more suitable for me, considering my health history and other medications I'm taking?
- What are the alternatives to statins for managing my cholesterol and reducing my risk of heart disease?
- If I decide to take statins, how will we monitor my progress and potential side effects?
- How can I safely discontinue statins if we decide they're no longer the right choice for me?
- What lifestyle changes can I make to support my heart health and potentially reduce my reliance on medication?

Safe Statin Discontinuation:

If you and your doctor decide that statins are no longer the right choice for you, it's essential to discontinue their use safely and gradually.

- **Never Abruptly Stop Taking Statins:** Suddenly stopping statins can lead to a rebound effect, causing your cholesterol levels to spike, potentially increasing your risk of heart problems.

- **Follow Your Doctor's Guidance:** Work closely with your doctor to develop a tapering schedule to gradually reduce your statin dosage over time. This allows your body to adjust and minimizes the risk of adverse effects.

- **Monitor Your Cholesterol Levels:** Your doctor will likely monitor your cholesterol levels closely during the discontinuation process to ensure your heart health is protected.

Your health journey is YOUR story, and you are the leading role. Taking charge means actively gathering information, having open conversations with your doctor, and speaking up about what you need. It's about making choices that feel right for you, aligned with your goals and values, not just accepting whatever's given.

The WARRIOR Approach: A Complementary Path to Wellness

Even if you and your doctor determine that statins are necessary for your heart health, embracing a holistic approach to wellness can complement your medical treatment, reduce your risk of side effects, and enhance your overall well-being. The WARRIOR approach emphasizes:

- **Reduced Inflammation:** Adopting an anti-inflammatory diet, managing stress, and incorporating gentle exercise can help reduce inflammation throughout your body, potentially minimizing statin-related muscle aches and supporting nerve health.

- **Enhanced Nutrition:** A nutrient-rich diet, focusing on whole, unprocessed foods and potentially incorporating targeted supplements like CoQ10, can support nerve health and mitigate the potential for statin-induced nutrient depletion.

- **Empowered Movement:** Regular, moderate-intensity exercise not only benefits your heart but also improves circulation, supports nerve function, and helps manage stress.

- **Whole-Body Wellness:** Addressing all aspects of your well-being—physical, emotional, and mental—can enhance your body's resilience, reduce your risk of side effects, and improve your overall quality of life.

As we've explored in this chapter, the decision to take statins is a deeply personal one, requiring careful consideration of both the potential benefits and risks. By understanding how statins work, their potential impact on nerve health, and the importance of individualized care, you can engage in informed conversations with your doctor and make choices that prioritize both your heart health and your overall well-being. Remember, a holistic approach to wellness, encompassing lifestyle modifications, a nutrient-rich diet, and stress management techniques, can empower you to take control of your health, reduce your risk of side effects, and create a vibrant foundation for a longer, healthier life.

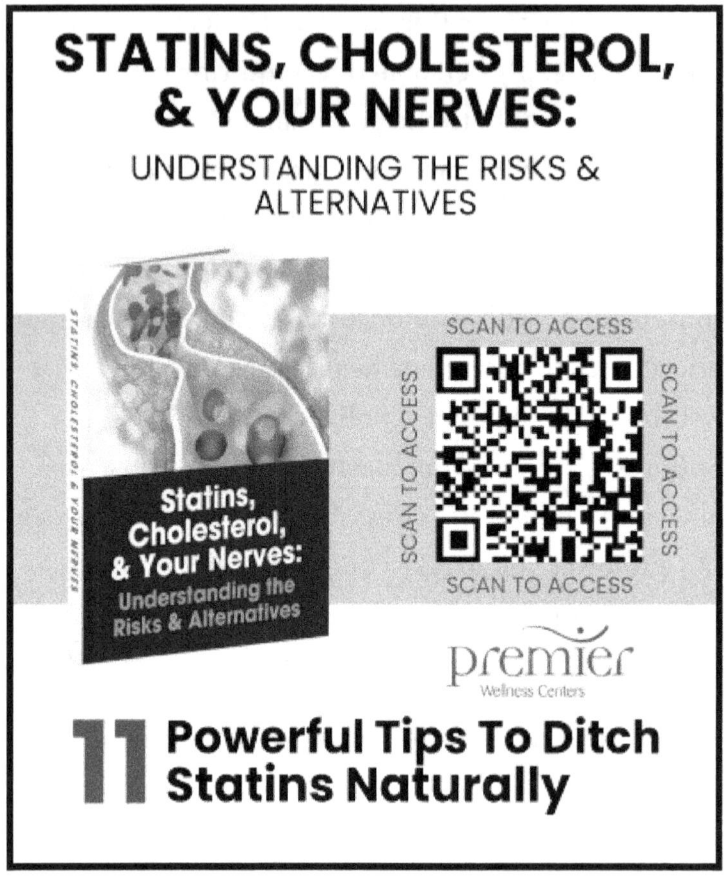

Unlock Your Path to Neuropathy Relief Now: Dial (772) 279-4145 to Speak With a Skilled Neuropathy Professional Today!

Individual results may vary. Please review the disclaimer after the Table of Contents.

10

THE GUT-NERVE CONNECTION: EXPLORING THE ROLE OF GLUTEN IN NEUROPATHY

Years ago, a patient named Karen came to see me with a baffling array of symptoms—fatigue, brain fog, digestive issues, and a persistent tingling in her hands and feet that had been diagnosed as peripheral neuropathy. We explored various possibilities, but nothing seemed to fully explain her complex web of health challenges.

Then, a lightbulb moment occurred during a conversation about her diet. Karen mentioned that she'd always felt worse after eating bread, pasta, or anything containing wheat. We decided to explore the possibility of gluten sensitivity, and I recommended she try an elimination diet, removing gluten from her diet for several weeks to see if her symptoms improved.

The transformation was remarkable. Within weeks, Karen's energy returned, the brain fog lifted, her digestion improved, and the tingling in her extremities significantly subsided. It was like a cloud had been lifted from her life. While we can't guarantee that everyone will experience the same benefits from a gluten-free diet, Karen's story highlights the profound connection between our gut and our nervous system.

It turns out that gluten, a protein found in wheat, rye, and barley, can trigger an immune response in some individuals, leading to inflammation that can damage nerves throughout the body. This connection, known as the gut-nerve axis, is a relatively new area of research, but it's shedding light on the often-overlooked role of gluten in contributing to neuropathy and other chronic health conditions.

Gluten: A Modern Dietary Dilemma

The allure of freshly baked bread, the siren call of pasta's comfort, and the whispered promise of a flaky croissant can be irresistible. But for those with gluten sensitivity, these delights can become a source of suffering. Gluten, the often-overlooked protein in these culinary masterpieces, can trigger a symphony of uncomfortable symptoms and even contribute to chronic health issues like neuropathy. This invisible foe presents a growing challenge to those navigating the world of food and health.

Gluten is a family of proteins found in wheat, rye, and barley. It gives dough its elasticity and chewy texture, making it a popular ingredient in a wide range of baked goods, pasta, cereals, and processed foods. For most people, gluten is harmlessly digested and poses no health threat. However, for those with gluten sensitivity or celiac disease, consuming gluten can spark an immune response that leads to inflammation in the gut and potentially throughout the body.

You might think gluten intolerance is all about a rumbling tummy and a trip to the bathroom. But recent research suggests there might be a lot more to it than that. Scientists are uncovering surprising connections between gluten sensitivity and a wider range of health issues. From autoimmune diseases that affect your entire body to skin problems, throbbing headaches, and even a fogginess in your thinking, it seems gluten could be pulling the strings on our well-being in ways we never imagined.

For individuals with neuropathy, understanding the potential role of gluten is crucial. It might be a hidden trigger, exacerbating symptoms or hindering healing. By exploring this connection, you can make informed decisions about your diet and potentially discover a path toward greater relief and improved nerve health.

Untangling the Terminology: Celiac Disease, Gluten Sensitivity, and Wheat Allergy

Navigating the world of gluten-related disorders can feel like trying to solve a complex puzzle. The terms "celiac disease," "gluten sensitivity," and "wheat allergy" are often used interchangeably, but they represent distinct conditions with different mechanisms, symptoms, and diagnostic criteria.

Here's a breakdown to help you understand the differences:

- **Celiac Disease: An Autoimmune Reaction**

You wouldn't expect something as common as wheat to unleash an autoimmune attack, but that's exactly what happens in celiac disease. The gluten protein found in wheat, rye, and barley, somehow sets off an inflammatory response that targets the villi, those vital finger-like structures in the small intestine responsible for nutrient absorption. It's an intriguing mystery how such a seemingly benign substance can trigger such a serious condition. Regardless, the impact can be significant, leading to digestive problems and nutrient deficiencies that impact overall health.

- **Gluten Sensitivity: A Spectrum of Reactions**

Gluten sensitivity throws a curveball, wreaking havoc on your well-being without a clear explanation. It's as if your body has a secret pact with gluten, whispering warnings of digestive distress, aching joints, and mental fog after even the smallest bite. While the mechanics behind this relationship remain under investigation, one thing's certain: it can take a toll on your daily life. This silent rebellion against gluten might not show up on a test, but its symptoms are real and demanding attention.

- **Wheat Allergy: A True Allergy**

A wheat allergy is a true allergic reaction to proteins found in wheat, including gluten. It triggers an immune response that releases histamine and other chemicals, leading to symptoms like hives, itching, swelling, difficulty breathing, and even anaphylaxis— a life-threatening allergic reaction.

Beyond the Gut: The Varied Manifestations of Gluten-Related Disorders

While gluten-related disorders are often associated with digestive problems, their effects can reach far beyond the gut, manifesting in surprising and often confusing ways. This is why getting an accurate diagnosis is crucial, as it guides appropriate treatment and helps prevent long-term health complications.

Here's a closer look at how each condition can present differently:

Celiac Disease: A Spectrum of Symptoms Beyond Digestion

While classic celiac disease often involves digestive symptoms like diarrhea, bloating, gas, and abdominal pain, it can also manifest in a wide range of seemingly unrelated ways:

- **Neurological Issues:** Celiac disease has been linked to an increased risk of neuropathy, as well as headaches, migraines, dizziness, and even seizures.
- **Skin Problems:** Some individuals with celiac disease develop dermatitis herpetiformis, an itchy, blistering skin rash.
- **Nutrient Deficiencies:** Damage to the small intestine can impair nutrient absorption, leading to deficiencies in iron, vitamin B12, folate, and other essential

nutrients. This can contribute to fatigue, anemia, bone loss, and other health problems.

- **Autoimmune Disorders:** Celiac disease is associated with an increased risk of other autoimmune disorders, such as thyroid disease and type 1 diabetes.

Gluten Sensitivity: A Diagnostic Challenge

Diagnosing gluten sensitivity can be tricky because its symptoms often overlap with other conditions, and there's no definitive blood test or biomarker. Symptoms can vary widely from person to person, often involving a combination of:

- **Digestive Problems:** Bloating, gas, diarrhea, constipation, abdominal pain, nausea.
- **Neurological Issues:** Headaches, migraines, brain fog, fatigue, difficulty concentrating, mood changes.
- **Joint and Muscle Pain:** Aches, stiffness, inflammation.
- **Skin Problems:** Eczema, acne, rashes.

Wheat Allergy: A Clear and Present Danger

Wheat allergy usually manifests as an immediate

allergic reaction after consuming wheat. Symptoms can range from mild to severe, including:

- **Skin Reactions:** Hives, itching, eczema.
- **Respiratory Problems:** Wheezing, coughing, difficulty breathing.
- **Gastrointestinal Issues:** Nausea, vomiting, diarrhea, abdominal cramps.
- **Anaphylaxis:** A life-threatening allergic reaction that can cause airway constriction, a drop in blood pressure, and even shock.

The Importance of Accurate Diagnosis

Getting an accurate diagnosis is crucial for several reasons:

- **Appropriate Treatment:** Each condition requires a specific approach. Celiac disease necessitates a lifelong gluten-free diet, while gluten sensitivity might involve a period of gluten elimination followed by careful reintroduction to assess tolerance. Wheat allergy requires strict avoidance of wheat and prompt medical attention in case of accidental exposure.
- **Preventing Complications:** Untreated celiac disease can lead to long-term health

complications, including malnutrition, osteoporosis, infertility, and an increased risk of certain cancers.

- **Improving Quality of Life:** By identifying the culprit behind your symptoms, you can make informed choices about your diet and lifestyle, potentially leading to significant symptom relief and improved quality of life.

Unmasking the Culprit: Testing for Gluten-Related Disorders

If you suspect you might have a gluten-related disorder, it's essential to seek professional guidance for proper testing and diagnosis. Here's a brief overview of the testing options available for each condition:

Celiac Disease: Blood Tests and Biopsy

- **Blood Tests:** Blood tests can detect antibodies that are produced in response to gluten in people with celiac disease. Common tests include tissue transglutaminase IgA (tTG IgA) and anti-endomysial antibodies (EMA).
- **Endoscopy and Biopsy:** If blood tests suggest celiac disease, your doctor might recommend

an endoscopy, a procedure in which a thin, flexible tube with a camera is inserted into your small intestine to examine the lining and take a small tissue sample (biopsy). The biopsy can confirm the presence of villous atrophy, a hallmark of celiac disease.

Gluten Sensitivity: A Diagnosis of Exclusion

Currently, there's no definitive test for gluten sensitivity. Diagnosis is often made through a process of exclusion, ruling out other conditions like celiac disease and wheat allergy.

- **Elimination Diet:** Your doctor might recommend eliminating gluten from your diet for several weeks to see if your symptoms improve.
- **Reintroduction Challenge:** If your symptoms improve on a gluten-free diet, your doctor might advise a carefully controlled reintroduction of gluten to assess your tolerance.

Wheat Allergy: Allergy Testing

- **Skin Prick Test:** This test involves placing a small amount of wheat protein extract on your skin and pricking the area with a needle. If you're allergic, a red, itchy bump (wheal) will appear.

- **Blood Test (RAST):** This test measures the amount of wheat-specific IgE antibodies in your blood, which indicates an allergic reaction.

Remember, these are just brief descriptions of common testing methods. Your doctor will determine the most appropriate tests based on your individual symptoms, medical history, and concerns.

Beyond Digestion: Unveiling the Gut-Brain-Nerve Connection

For years, we viewed the gut and the brain as separate entities, each responsible for distinct functions. However, groundbreaking research is revealing a fascinating and intricate connection between these two seemingly disparate systems—a link so profound that it's been dubbed the "gut-brain axis." What's more, this intricate connection extends to our nerves, playing a potential role in the development and progression of neuropathy.

The Gut-Brain Superhighway:

Imagine a bustling two-way highway, with a constant flow of information traveling between your gut and your brain. That's essentially how the gut-brain axis operates. It's a complex communication network involving:

- **The Vagus Nerve:** This long nerve acts as a direct communication pathway between the gut and the brain, carrying signals in both directions.
- **Neurotransmitters:** These chemical messengers, produced in both the gut and the brain, influence mood, cognition, and even pain perception.
- **The Immune System:** A significant portion of your immune system resides in your gut, and its activity can influence inflammation throughout the body, including in the nervous system.

The Microbiome: Your Gut's Inner Ecosystem

Your gut is home to trillions of bacteria, fungi, and other microorganisms collectively known as your gut microbiome. This internal ecosystem plays a far greater role in our overall health than we previously understood.

- **Influencing Digestion:** Gut bacteria help break down food, extract nutrients, and synthesize vitamins.
- **Shaping Immunity:** The gut microbiome interacts with your immune system, influencing its development and activity.
- **Impacting the Brain:** Emerging evidence suggests that the gut microbiome can influence brain function, mood, and even behavior.

The Gluten-Neuropathy Puzzle: Connecting the Dots

While the exact mechanisms by which gluten impacts nerve health are still being investigated, research suggests several potential pathways:

- **Immune Activation and Inflammation:** In individuals with gluten sensitivity or celiac disease, consuming gluten triggers an immune response that leads to inflammation in the gut. This inflammation, if chronic, can extend beyond the digestive system, affecting nerves throughout the body.

- **Leaky Gut and Increased Permeability:** Gluten might contribute to increased intestinal permeability, often referred to as "leaky gut," allowing undigested food particles, toxins, and bacteria to leak into the bloodstream. This can trigger inflammation and immune activation, potentially damaging nerves.

- **Nutrient Malabsorption:** Inflammation and damage to the small intestine in celiac disease can impair nutrient absorption, leading to deficiencies that can contribute to neuropathy, particularly deficiencies in B vitamins, which are crucial for nerve health.

This intricate gut-brain-nerve connection underscores a crucial point: our digestive health is intricately intertwined with our neurological well-being. By nurturing a healthy gut microbiome through dietary choices, stress management, and other lifestyle modifications, we can potentially reduce inflammation, support nerve health, and enhance overall well-being.

Gluten Under Fire: How It Triggers Nerve Damage

While the connection between gluten and neuropathy is complex and still being fully elucidated, research suggests several mechanisms by which this dietary protein can wreak havoc on our delicate nervous system.

1. Immune System Activation: A Cascade of Inflammation

For individuals with gluten sensitivity or celiac disease, consuming gluten triggers an immune response in the gut. Think of it like an internal alarm system going haywire, sending out inflammatory troops to attack a perceived threat—in this case, gluten. This inflammatory cascade, while intended to protect the body, can damage the lining of the small intestine and, in some cases, extend beyond the gut, affecting nerves throughout the body.

Imagine a fire breaking out in a building. The initial flames might be contained to one room, but if left unchecked, they can spread rapidly, causing damage throughout the structure. Similarly, chronic inflammation triggered by gluten can damage the delicate myelin sheath that insulates nerve fibers, disrupting nerve signaling and leading to those familiar neuropathy symptoms—tingling, numbness, pain, and weakness.

2. Nutrient Malabsorption: Starving Your Nerves

The inflammatory damage to the small intestine in celiac disease can impair the absorption of vital nutrients, including those essential for nerve health. B vitamins, in particular, play a crucial role in nerve cell function, repair, and the production of neurotransmitters—the chemical messengers that allow nerves to communicate.

Imagine your nerves as delicate plants that need a steady supply of water and nutrients to thrive. When gluten-related inflammation disrupts nutrient absorption, it's like depriving those plants of essential nourishment, leading to their weakening, dysfunction, and eventual "withering"—manifesting as neuropathy symptoms.

3. Leaky Gut: Breaching the Barriers

Gluten has been implicated in increasing intestinal permeability—often referred to as "leaky gut." Imagine the lining of your gut as a finely woven net, carefully controlling what passes from your digestive system into your bloodstream. Gluten, in susceptible individuals, can disrupt the integrity of this net, creating gaps that allow undigested food particles, toxins, and bacteria to leak into the bloodstream.

This breach in the gut barrier triggers a systemic immune response, as your body tries to defend itself against these foreign invaders. This widespread inflammation can damage nerves throughout the body, contributing to the development or worsening of neuropathy.

These interconnected mechanisms highlight the profound impact gluten can have on our nervous system, particularly in those with a sensitivity or intolerance. By understanding these pathways, we can make informed choices about our diet and potentially mitigate the risk of gluten-induced nerve damage.

Connecting the Dots: Scientific Evidence Linking Gluten and Neuropathy

While more research is always needed, a growing body of scientific evidence suggests a strong link between gluten sensitivity and various forms of neuropathy. Let's delve into some key studies that shed light on this connection:

The Prevalence of Gluten-Related Neuropathy:

- **Neuropathy in Celiac Patients:** A study published in the journal *Acta Neurologica Scandinavica* examined the prevalence of neuropathy in individuals with confirmed celiac disease who were already following a gluten-free diet. The study revealed a surprisingly high occurrence, with 23% of these individuals showing evidence of axonal peripheral neuropathy, indicating damage to the long nerve fibers that transmit signals throughout the body [1].

- **Varied Prevalence, Consistent Risk:** A comprehensive review of multiple studies, published in *Nutrients,* found that the reported prevalence of gluten-related neuropathy in celiac patients varied across studies, likely due to differences in diagnostic criteria and study populations. However, the review consistently highlighted an increased risk of neuropathy in those with celiac disease, emphasizing the need for further research to better understand this connection [2].

The Power of a Gluten-Free Diet:

- **Symptom Improvement on a Gluten-Free Diet:** A prospective study involving 35 patients with gluten neuropathy, published in *Nutrients,* provided compelling evidence for the benefits of dietary intervention. Twenty-five of these patients were instructed to adhere strictly to a gluten-free diet, while the remaining ten served as a control group. The results were striking: 16 out of the 25 patients on the gluten-free diet reported significant improvement in their neuropathy symptoms, while none of the patients in the control group experienced any improvement [2].

- **Reduced Pain with Dietary Adherence:** A study presented at the American Academy of Neurology's 68th Annual Meeting in 2016 examined the relationship between gluten-free diet adherence and neuropathy pain. After adjusting for factors like age, gender, and mental health status, the researchers discovered a remarkable finding: individuals who strictly followed a gluten-free diet were 89% less likely to experience pain associated with their neuropathy compared to those who did not follow the diet [3].

- **Neurophysiological Improvement:** A case-control study published in *ScienceDirect* demonstrated that a gluten-free diet led to improvements in neurophysiological measures—objective assessments of nerve function—as well as a reduction in neuropathy symptoms in patients with gluten sensitivity [4].

Unraveling the Mechanisms:

While the exact mechanisms by which gluten triggers neuropathy are still being investigated, research suggests an immune-mediated process, similar to that seen in gluten ataxia, a neurological condition affecting balance and coordination.

- **Inflammatory Assault on Nerves:** The prevailing theory is that gluten, in susceptible individuals, triggers an inflammatory response that can damage both peripheral nerves and the central nervous system [1].

These studies, along with others emerging in the field, provide compelling evidence for the link between gluten sensitivity and neuropathy. While more research is always needed to fully understand the complex interplay of factors, these findings offer hope for those seeking to manage their neuropathy symptoms. A gluten-free diet, in conjunction with other appropriate therapies, might offer a path toward relief and improved nerve health.

Citations:

[1] https://www.ncbi.nlm.nih.gov/pmc/articles/PMC2077388/

[2] https://www.ncbi.nlm.nih.gov/pmc/articles/PMC6412791/

[3] https://www.aan.com/Press-Room/Home/PressRelease/1627

[4] https://www.sciencedirect.com/topics/immunology-and-microbiology/gluten-sensitivity

Gluten's Reach: Types of Neuropathy Linked to Sensitivity

While more research is needed to fully understand the complex relationship between gluten and nerve damage, studies have linked gluten sensitivity to several types of neuropathy:

- **Peripheral Neuropathy:** This is the most common type associated with gluten sensitivity. It affects the nerves in the extremities—the hands, feet, arms, and legs—leading to symptoms like tingling, numbness, pain, and weakness.
- **Small Fiber Neuropathy:** This type affects the small nerve fibers responsible for

transmitting pain and temperature sensations. It often causes burning pain, particularly in the feet, and can also affect autonomic functions like sweating and heart rate. Gluten sensitivity has been implicated as a potential trigger for this often-painful form of neuropathy.

- **Autonomic Neuropathy:** While less common than peripheral neuropathy, some studies suggest a potential link between gluten sensitivity and autonomic neuropathy, which affects the nerves that control involuntary bodily functions like heart rate, blood pressure, digestion, and bladder function.
- **Gluten Ataxia:** This neurological condition affects balance and coordination, often causing a stumbling gait, difficulty with fine motor skills, and slurred speech. While gluten ataxia primarily affects the cerebellum (the part of the brain responsible for coordination), it can also involve peripheral nerve damage.

It's important to note that gluten sensitivity is not the sole cause of these types of neuropathy. Many other factors can contribute, including diabetes, autoimmune disorders, vitamin deficiencies, and exposure to toxins. However, gluten sensitivity can be a significant contributing factor in some cases, and identifying this connection can be crucial for effective treatment and symptom management.

From Gluten-Free to Symptom-Free: Case Studies in Healing

While large-scale studies provide valuable insights into the link between gluten and neuropathy, real-life case studies offer compelling evidence of the transformative power of a gluten-free diet for those struggling with nerve-related symptoms. Here are a few examples that highlight the potential for healing:

- **Motor Neuropathy: Regaining Strength and Function:** A study published in *Cureus* followed two individuals with motor-predominant neuropathy—a type of neuropathy that primarily affects muscle strength and control—associated with biopsy-proven celiac disease [1]. Both patients showed remarkable improvement in their strength, nerve function (as measured by nerve conduction studies), and even intestinal health after adopting a strict gluten-free diet. This case is particularly striking because one of the patients had previously received intravenous immunoglobulin (IVIG) therapy, a common treatment for autoimmune neuropathy, with no noticeable benefit. However, simply eliminating gluten from their diet led to significant improvement.

- **Sensory Ganglionopathy: Halting Progression with Dietary Change:** A study published in *Cureus* examined 17 patients with sensory ganglionopathy, a type of neuropathy that affects the sensory nerves, and gluten sensitivity [1]. Eleven of these patients adhered strictly to a gluten-free diet and experienced stable symptoms, meaning their neuropathy did not worsen. However, the six patients who either did not adhere to the diet or did not participate at all experienced progressive symptoms, indicating a worsening of their neuropathy. This case highlights the importance of strict dietary adherence for managing gluten-related neuropathy.

- **Clear Improvement with Strict Adherence:** A systematic study published in *Neurosurgical Focus* examined the effects of a gluten-free diet in a large group of patients with gluten neuropathy [2]. The study demonstrated clear clinical and neurophysiological improvement after 12 months in those who adhered strictly to the diet, reinforcing the link between dietary intervention and symptom reduction.

- **Small Fiber Neuropathy: Relief from Burning Pain:** A case series published in *JAMA Neurology* involved four patients with small fiber neuropathy and celiac disease, a condition known to be strongly associated with gluten intolerance [4]. All four patients reported improvement in their neuropathy symptoms, including a reduction in the often-debilitating burning pain that characterizes this type of neuropathy, after adopting a gluten-free diet.
- **Neurophysiological and Symptom Improvement:** A case-control study published in *ScienceDirect* demonstrated that a gluten-free diet led to improvements in neurophysiological measures—objective assessments of nerve function—as well as a reduction in neuropathy symptoms in patients with gluten sensitivity [3].

These cases, while not representative of everyone's experience, provide compelling evidence that a gluten-free diet can be a powerful tool for managing and relieving neuropathy symptoms in individuals with gluten sensitivity. While not all patients experience the same level of improvement, and some might face challenges with strict dietary adherence or irreversible nerve damage, these stories offer hope and highlight the potential for positive change through dietary intervention.

Citations:

[1] https://www.ncbi.nlm.nih.gov/pmc/articles/PMC8485976/

[2] https://link.springer.com/article/10.1007/s11940-019-0552-7

[3] https://www.sciencedirect.com/topics/immunology-and-microbiology/gluten-sensitivity

[4] https://jamanetwork.com/journals/jamaneurology/fullarticle/789587

Navigating the Gluten-Free World: A Practical Guide to Getting Started

Embarking on a gluten-free journey can feel overwhelming at first, especially when gluten seems to lurk in so many foods we love. But with a little knowledge and planning, it's entirely possible to make the transition smoothly and enjoy a delicious and satisfying gluten-free lifestyle.

Here's a step-by-step guide to help you get started:

1. Become a Label Detective: Unveiling Hidden Gluten

Gluten is a master of disguise, often hiding in unexpected places. Learning to read food labels carefully is crucial for avoiding accidental gluten exposure.

- **The Obvious Culprits:** Look for obvious sources of gluten, like wheat, rye, and barley, listed in the ingredients.
- **Hidden Gluten Hotspots:** Gluten can sneak into a surprising range of processed foods, including:
  - **Sauces and Condiments:** Soy sauce, salad dressings, marinades, gravy.
  - **Processed Meats:** Sausages, hot dogs, deli meats.
  - **Soup and Broth:** Many commercially prepared soups and broths contain gluten as a thickener.
  - **Snacks and Sweets:** Candy, chocolate, granola bars, chips, crackers.

- ○ **Flavorings and Additives:** Malt flavoring, modified food starch, hydrolyzed vegetable protein.
- **Look for "Gluten-Free" Certification:** Seek out products labeled "gluten-free," which indicates they meet strict standards for gluten content.

Tips for Success:

- **Start Simple:** Don't try to overhaul your entire diet overnight. Begin by gradually replacing gluten-containing foods with naturally gluten-free options, like fruits, vegetables, lean proteins, and healthy fats.
- **Stock Your Pantry:** Keep your kitchen stocked with gluten-free staples, like rice, quinoa, gluten-free oats, nuts, seeds, beans, lentils, and plenty of fresh produce.
- **Read Labels Every Time:** Even if you think you know a product is gluten-free, always double-check the label, as ingredients can change.
- **Ask Questions When Dining Out:** Don't hesitate to ask about gluten-free options when dining out. Many restaurants now offer

gluten-free menus or can modify dishes to accommodate your dietary needs.

- **Join a Support Group or Online Community:** Connecting with others on a gluten-free journey can provide valuable support, recipes, and tips for navigating the transition.

Remember, going gluten-free is a process. Be patient with yourself, celebrate small victories, and don't be afraid to experiment in the kitchen to discover delicious and satisfying gluten-free meals that nourish your body and support your health.

Beyond Wheat and Rye: Embracing Gluten-Free Deliciousness

Going gluten-free doesn't mean sacrificing flavor, variety, or satisfaction. There's a whole world of naturally gluten-free grains, flours, and delicious substitutes just waiting to be explored. It's an opportunity to expand your culinary horizons, discover new favorites, and nourish your body with a rainbow of flavors.

Gluten-Free Grains and Flours:

- **Rice:** A versatile staple, rice comes in various forms   white, brown, wild, and even black—

offering a range of textures and flavors to suit any dish.

- **Quinoa:** This protein-packed ancient grain is a complete protein, meaning it contains all nine essential amino acids. It has a slightly nutty flavor and cooks up quickly.

- **Oats (Certified Gluten-Free):** Oats are naturally gluten-free but are often cross-contaminated with gluten during processing. Look for certified gluten-free oats to ensure they're safe for your dietary needs.

- **Millet:** This ancient grain is a good source of fiber, iron, and magnesium. It has a mild, slightly sweet flavor and can be used in porridges, salads, or as a side dish.

- **Corn:** From tortillas to polenta to cornmeal, corn is a versatile gluten-free grain that can be enjoyed in countless ways.

- **Buckwheat:** Despite its name, buckwheat is not related to wheat and is naturally gluten-free. It has a nutty, earthy flavor and can be used in pancakes, soba noodles, or as a hearty salad base.

Flour Power: Gluten-Free Baking

- **Almond Flour:** Made from finely ground almonds, almond flour is a popular gluten-free alternative that adds a subtle nuttiness and richness to baked goods.
- **Coconut Flour:** Made from dried coconut meat, coconut flour is high in fiber and adds a slightly sweet flavor to recipes. It tends to absorb more liquid than other flours, so recipes often require additional eggs or liquid.
- **Tapioca Flour:** Made from the cassava root, tapioca flour is a grain-free option that adds a chewy texture to baked goods. It's often used as a thickener in soups and sauces.
- **Gluten-Free All-Purpose Blends:** Many commercially prepared gluten-free all-purpose flour blends combine various gluten-free flours and starches to create a versatile option for baking.

Focusing on Nutrient Density:

While gluten-free substitutes can make the transition easier, the real key to a healthy gluten-free diet is focusing on whole, unprocessed foods.

- **Fruits and Vegetables:** Fill your plate with a rainbow of colorful fruits and vegetables, which provide a wealth of vitamins, minerals, antioxidants, and fiber.
- **Lean Proteins:** Choose lean protein sources, like chicken, fish, turkey, beans, lentils, and tofu, to support muscle mass and overall health.
- **Healthy Fats:** Incorporate healthy fats, like those found in avocados, olive oil, nuts, and fatty fish, to support nerve health, reduce inflammation, and enhance nutrient absorption.
- **Mindful Eating:** Pay attention to your hunger and fullness cues, and savor each bite to enhance digestion and satisfaction.

Gluten-Free and Delicious: Meal Planning Made Easy

Transitioning to a gluten-free diet doesn't have to be a culinary upheaval. With a little planning and a sprinkle of creativity, you can enjoy delicious, satisfying meals that nourish your body and support your health.

Here's a sample meal plan and a simple recipe to inspire your gluten-free journey:

Sample Gluten-Free Meal Plan:

- **Breakfast:** Start your day with a blood-sugar-balancing and nutrient-rich breakfast:
    - **Option 1:** Smoothie made with unsweetened almond milk, spinach, berries, a scoop of protein powder, and chia seeds.
    - **Option 2:** Scrambled eggs with sautéed vegetables (onions, peppers, spinach) and a side of avocado.
    - **Option 3:** Gluten-free oatmeal topped with berries, nuts, and a drizzle of honey or maple syrup.
- **Lunch:** Keep your energy levels stable and nourish your body with these satisfying lunch ideas:
    - **Option 1:** Big salad with grilled chicken or fish, quinoa, roasted vegetables, and a light vinaigrette dressing.
    - **Option 2:** Lentil soup with a side of gluten-free bread and a mixed green salad.
    - **Option 3:** Leftovers from dinner!
- **Dinner:** End your day with a delicious and nourishing gluten-free meal:

- o **Option 1:** Baked salmon with roasted Brussels sprouts and a side of wild rice.
  - o **Option 2:** Chicken and vegetable stir-fry served over brown rice or cauliflower rice.
  - o **Option 3:** Turkey meatballs with zucchini noodles and marinara sauce.
- **Snacks:** Keep healthy, gluten-free snacks on hand to prevent blood sugar dips and nourish your body between meals:
  - o A handful of pistachios or walnuts
  - o A piece of fruit with a tablespoon of nut butter
  - o Carrot sticks or celery sticks with hummus
  - o Plain coconut yogurt with berries and a sprinkle of cinnamon

Recipe Inspiration: Simple and Satisfying Gluten-Free Pancakes

These fluffy, delicious pancakes are perfect for a comforting breakfast or brunch.

Ingredients:

- 1 cup gluten-free all-purpose flour
- 1 teaspoon baking powder

- 1/2 teaspoon baking soda
- 1/4 teaspoon salt
- 1 tablespoon sugar
- 1 egg
- 1 cup milk (dairy or non-dairy)
- 2 tablespoons melted butter or coconut oil

Instructions:

1. In a large bowl, whisk together the flour, baking powder, baking soda, salt, and sugar.
2. In a separate bowl, whisk together the egg, milk, and melted butter or coconut oil.
3. Pour the wet ingredients into the dry ingredients and whisk until just combined. Don't overmix.
4. Heat a lightly greased griddle or skillet over medium heat.
5. Pour 1/4 cup of batter onto the hot griddle for each pancake.
6. Cook for 2-3 minutes per side, or until golden brown and cooked through.
7. Serve with your favorite toppings, like fresh fruit, maple syrup, or nut butter.

Now this is just a starting point. There are endless possibilities for creating delicious and satisfying gluten-free meals. Explore new recipes, experiment with different gluten-free ingredients, and embrace the joy of cooking and eating nourishing foods that support your health and well-being.

The Gluten-Free Journey: Beyond the Basics

While eliminating gluten can be a game-changer for many individuals with neuropathy, it's essential to remember that it's not a one-size-fits-all solution, and there are other important factors to consider for long-term success.

Seek Personalized Guidance from Healthcare Professionals:

Navigating dietary changes, especially when you have underlying health conditions, is best done in partnership with knowledgeable healthcare professionals.

- **Consult with Your Doctor:** Discuss your concerns about gluten and neuropathy with your doctor. We can help determine if gluten sensitivity is a potential contributor to your symptoms and order appropriate tests to rule out celiac disease or other conditions.
- **Partner with a Registered Dietitian:** A registered dietitian specializing in gluten-free

diets can provide personalized guidance, create a tailored meal plan, and ensure you're meeting your nutritional needs while avoiding gluten.

Unmasking Other Dietary Culprits:

Gluten is not the only dietary trigger for neuropathy. Other foods can contribute to inflammation, nerve damage, and symptom flare-ups.

- **Common Food Sensitivities:** Dairy, soy, eggs, corn, and nightshades (tomatoes, potatoes, peppers) are common culprits behind food sensitivities that can trigger inflammation and worsen neuropathy symptoms.
- **Elimination Diet:** If you suspect other food sensitivities, discuss an elimination diet with your healthcare provider or a registered dietitian. This involves temporarily removing certain foods from your diet and then gradually reintroducing them one at a time to identify any triggers.

Sustainable Changes for Lasting Health:

Going gluten-free shouldn't feel like a restrictive diet; it's an opportunity to embrace a wide range of delicious and nourishing foods that support your overall health and well-being.

- **Focus on Whole Foods:** Prioritize whole, unprocessed foods, such as fruits, vegetables, lean proteins, healthy fats, and gluten-free grains. These foods provide the nutrients your body needs to thrive and help reduce inflammation.
- **Experiment with New Flavors:** Explore the world of gluten-free grains, flours, and recipes. Don't be afraid to get creative in the kitchen and discover new favorites.
- **Make It a Lifestyle:** View going gluten-free not as a temporary fix but as a long-term lifestyle change that supports your overall health and helps manage your neuropathy.

Taking Charge: Your Gluten-Free Path to Neuropathy Relief

As we've explored in this chapter, the connection between gluten and neuropathy is complex and multifaceted. While gluten is a harmless protein for most people, it can trigger a cascade of inflammatory reactions in those with gluten sensitivity or celiac disease, potentially leading to nerve damage and a worsening of neuropathy symptoms.

It's crucial to remember that a gluten-free diet is not a magic bullet for neuropathy. It's not a guaranteed cure for everyone. However, scientific evidence and real-life case studies suggest that eliminating gluten can significantly improve neuropathy symptoms and overall well-being for many individuals, particularly those with a confirmed sensitivity to this common dietary protein.

If you suspect that gluten might be contributing to your neuropathy, don't hesitate to seek guidance from experienced healthcare professionals, like our team at PWC. We can help you:

- **Determine if gluten sensitivity is a factor in your neuropathy.**
- **Rule out other conditions, such as celiac disease or wheat allergy.**
- **Develop a personalized plan to manage your neuropathy, including dietary modifications, lifestyle changes, and targeted therapies.**
- **Provide support and guidance as you navigate the transition to a gluten-free lifestyle.**

Knowledge is power, and informed decision-making is key to reclaiming your health. By partnering with a healthcare team that understands the complexities of neuropathy and the potential role of gluten, you can take charge of your health journey, explore all available options, and create a path toward lasting relief, improved nerve function, and a brighter, healthier future.

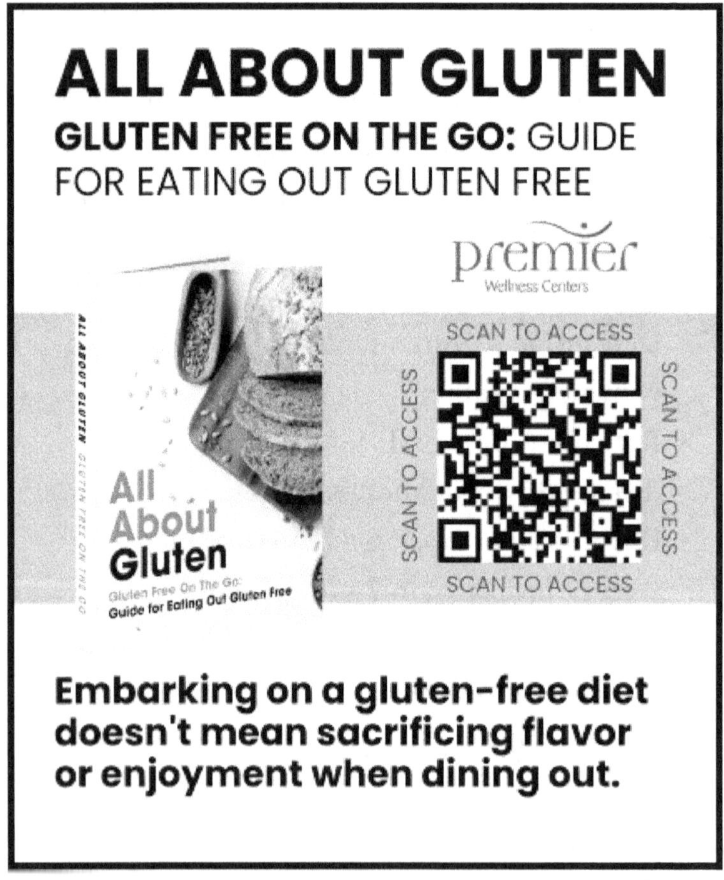

Unlock Your Path to Neuropathy Relief Now: Dial

(772) 279-4145 to Speak With a Skilled Neuropathy Professional Today!

Individual results may vary. Please review the disclaimer after the Table of Contents.

11

OPIOIDS AND NEUROPATHY: A RISKY EQUATION FOR PAIN RELIEF

The opioid crisis is not simply a statistic – it's a human tragedy playing out in countless homes and lives across our nation. What started with good intentions – a promise of pain relief – has been hijacked, twisted into a cruel addiction cycle fueled by the careless over-prescription of powerful drugs like oxycodone and the shadow world of heroin. Opioids have a legitimate place in medicine, capable of easing the most unbearable pain, but the very properties that make them effective in treating acute pain also make them dangerous, addictive, and vulnerable to misuse. When used long-term for chronic pain conditions, opioids pose significant risks:

- **Tolerance and Dependence:** Over time, the body develops a tolerance to opioids, requiring higher and higher doses to achieve the same level of pain relief. This can lead to physical dependence, where the body relies on the drug to function normally, and withdrawal symptoms occur when the drug is stopped.
- **Addiction:** Opioids have a high potential for addiction, even when used as prescribed. Addiction is a chronic, relapsing brain disease characterized by compulsive drug seeking and use, despite harmful consequences.
- **Overdose:** Opioid overdose occurs when the drug suppresses the respiratory system, leading to slowed breathing, loss of consciousness, and even death. The risk of overdose is significantly increased when opioids are combined with alcohol or other sedating medications.

This crisis intersects with neuropathy in a particularly challenging way. Neuropathy, as we know, is often characterized by chronic pain—relentless tingling, burning, stabbing sensations that can severely impact quality of life. In the past, opioids were often prescribed to manage this pain, leading to a cycle of dependence and, for some, a devastating spiral into addiction.

Opioids: A Double-Edged Sword of Pain Relief

To understand the risks and limitations of opioids for neuropathy, it's helpful to grasp how these powerful medications work on a cellular level.

Imagine your body as a vast communication network, with nerves acting like wires transmitting messages throughout your system. When you experience pain, those messages are sent from the site of injury or irritation, traveling along your nerves to your spinal cord and ultimately to your brain, where they're interpreted as pain.

Opioids step in to intercept these pain signals. They bind to specific receptors in your brain, spinal cord, and other parts of your body, essentially blocking the transmission of those pain messages. It's like flipping a switch to turn off the alarm system, preventing those pain signals from reaching their destination—your conscious awareness.

This ability to effectively block pain makes opioids valuable tools for managing acute pain, such as:

- **Post-Surgical Pain:** Opioids can help manage the intense pain often experienced after surgery, allowing for more comfortable recovery.
- **Trauma-Related Pain:** Opioids can provide much-needed relief for pain caused by injuries, such as fractures, burns, or severe wounds.
- **Cancer Pain:** Opioids are often used to manage the often-severe pain associated with cancer and its treatments.

However, while opioids can be lifesavers in these acute pain situations, their effectiveness for chronic pain conditions like neuropathy is limited, and their risks often outweigh their potential benefits.

The Opioid Family: From Prescription Painkillers to Illicit Drugs

Opioids encompass a wide range of substances, both legal and illegal, all sharing a common mechanism of action: they bind to opioid receptors in the body, blocking pain signals and producing feelings of euphoria.

Here's a look at some common types of opioids:

1. Prescription Painkillers:

These are opioids prescribed by doctors to manage pain, typically after surgery, injury, or for chronic pain conditions. Common examples include:

- **Oxycodone (OxyContin, Percocet):** A potent opioid often prescribed for moderate to severe pain.
- **Hydrocodone (Vicodin, Norco):** Another commonly prescribed opioid for moderate pain.
- **Morphine (MS Contin, Kadian):** A powerful opioid used to manage severe pain, often in hospital settings.
- **Codeine:** A weaker opioid often used in cough syrups or combined with other pain relievers.

2. Illegal Opioids:

Heroin is an illegal opioid synthesized from morphine. It's a highly addictive substance that poses serious health risks, including overdose and death.

3. Synthetic Opioids:

Imagine a painkiller so potent it's 50 to 100 times stronger than morphine. That's fentanyl, a synthetic opioid originally intended to help those battling excruciating pain, like cancer patients. But the darkness of the illicit drug market has hijacked its potential. Illegally manufactured fentanyl has become a silent killer, lurking within heroin and other drugs, making an overdose a horrifying possibility.

It's important to remember that even legitimate prescriptions, like any powerful medicine, come with risks. Used for prolonged periods or taken inappropriately, they can create a dangerous cycle of tolerance, dependence, and ultimately, addiction. Always follow your doctor's instructions and speak openly about your concerns – both about potential side effects and the real threat of addiction.

A Misguided Approach: Why Opioids Often Fail Neuropathy

In the past, opioids were commonly prescribed for neuropathic pain—the often relentless burning, tingling, and shooting pain that characterizes nerve damage. This practice, however, has come under intense scrutiny as we've gained a deeper understanding of neuropathy's complex mechanisms and the significant risks associated with long-term opioid use.

Here's why opioids are often a misguided approach for neuropathy pain:

- **Opioids Don't Address the Root Cause:** Opioids work by blocking pain signals in the brain, but they don't address the underlying nerve damage that causes neuropathic pain. It's like silencing the smoke alarm without putting out the fire—it might temporarily mask the problem, but the underlying damage continues to fester.

- **Diminishing Returns: The Tolerance Trap:** Over time, the body develops a tolerance to opioids, requiring higher and higher doses to achieve the same level of pain relief. This can lead to a dangerous cycle of increasing doses, increasing side effects, and diminishing returns, with the pain often returning as soon as the medication wears off.

- **A Recipe for Dependence and Addiction:** Neuropathic pain is often chronic, lasting for months or even years. Long-term opioid use for chronic pain carries a high risk of dependence and addiction, potentially leading to a devastating cycle of drug seeking and use, despite harmful consequences.

- **Exacerbating the Problem: Opioid-Induced Hyperalgesia:** In a cruel twist of irony, opioids can sometimes worsen pain in some individuals, a phenomenon known as opioid-induced hyperalgesia. This occurs because opioids can alter pain pathways in the brain and spinal cord, making individuals more sensitive to pain stimuli.

- **Side Effects That Compound Suffering:** Opioids come with a long list of potential side effects, many of which can significantly impact quality of life, including constipation, drowsiness, nausea, dizziness, cognitive impairment, and respiratory depression. These side effects can further complicate the challenges of living with neuropathy.

This complex relationship between opioids and neuropathy highlights a crucial shift in the approach to managing nerve-related pain. Instead of relying on opioids as a first-line treatment, the focus has shifted towards safer, more effective, and sustainable approaches that address the root causes of neuropathy and prioritize long-term healing and well-being.

Unmasking the Limitations: Why Opioids Often Fail Neuropathy

While opioids can effectively block pain signals in the brain, their effectiveness for long-term management of neuropathy is limited, and their risks often outweigh their potential benefits. This is because neuropathic pain—the pain arising from nerve damage—differs from other types of pain and doesn't respond predictably to opioids.

Here's a closer look at why opioids fall short for neuropathy:

- **Neuropathic Pain: A Different Beast:** Neuropathic pain is often described as burning, tingling, shooting, or electric shock-like sensations. It arises from damage to the nerves themselves, rather than from tissue injury or inflammation. Opioids, while effective for nociceptive pain (pain from tissue damage), often fail to adequately address the unique mechanisms underlying neuropathic pain.
- **The Tolerance Trap: Chasing Diminishing Returns:** Your body can get used to opioid painkillers. It's like a game of catch-up – each time, you need a bigger dose to feel the same

relief. This can turn into a harmful cycle. As the doses go up, you might experience more side effects, but the pain relief weakens, and your pain often returns quickly when the medication wears off.

- **Dependence and Addiction: A Slippery Slope:** Neuropathic pain can feel like a relentless shadow, haunting you for months, even years on end. Unfortunately, relying on opioids for long-term relief comes with a hefty price tag: dependence and addiction. Dependence, in a nutshell, means your body becomes so accustomed to the drug that it practically demands it. Stop the opioids, and you'll face uncomfortable withdrawal symptoms. Addiction, a much deeper and trickier beast, is like a tangled web you get trapped in. The brain, taken hostage by this craving, compels you to seek the drug no matter the consequences, turning a desperate desire for pain relief into a potentially life-altering addiction.

- **A Cascade of Side Effects:** Opioids are notorious for their side effects, many of which can significantly impair quality of life and exacerbate the challenges of living with neuropathy:

- Constipation: Opioids slow down the digestive system, leading to constipation, which can be uncomfortable and, in severe cases, even dangerous.
- Drowsiness and Cognitive Impairment: Opioids can cause drowsiness, dizziness, and difficulty concentrating, making it challenging to work, drive, or engage in daily activities.
- Nausea and Vomiting: Opioids can trigger nausea and vomiting, particularly in those new to the medication.
- Respiratory Depression: In high doses, opioids can suppress the respiratory system, leading to slowed breathing, a potentially life-threatening condition.

- **The Paradox of Opioid-Induced Hyperalgesia:** In some cases, opioids can paradoxically worsen pain, a phenomenon known as opioid-induced hyperalgesia. This occurs because opioids can alter pain pathways in the brain and spinal cord, increasing sensitivity to pain stimuli.

This complex interplay of factors underscores the need for a more nuanced approach to managing neuropathy pain—one that addresses the root causes, considers the unique mechanisms of neuropathic pain, and prioritizes safer, more effective, and sustainable solutions.

A Holistic Path to Pain Relief

We've learned a hard lesson about the dangers of long-term opioid use, especially for conditions like neuropathy that plague us for years. The old "mask the pain and move on" strategy has thankfully given way to a more intelligent, patient-centered approach. Now, doctors are focusing on getting to the heart of the problem, taking into account the unique circumstances of each individual, and recommending safer, more lasting solutions. This shift signifies a welcome departure from simply treating the symptoms and delving into the complex reality of chronic pain.

The Power of a Multidisciplinary Team:

Neuropathy is a complex condition, but with the right care team, managing it becomes a whole lot easier. Doctors, therapists, and even counselors work together to understand your needs and design a treatment plan that feels uniquely suited to you. This multidisciplinary approach, like the building blocks of a sturdy house, addresses your physical, emotional, and mental well-being, making your journey through neuropathy smoother and more hopeful.

Here are some key members who might be involved in your neuropathy care:

- **Chiropractor:** Chiropractors specialize in the diagnosis and treatment of musculoskeletal disorders, often employing spinal adjustments, manual therapies, and other techniques to alleviate pain, improve nerve function, and restore mobility.
- **Physical Therapist:** A physical therapist can help you regain strength, flexibility, balance, and coordination through targeted exercises and therapeutic modalities.
- **Acupuncturist:** Acupuncture, a traditional Chinese medicine practice, involves inserting thin needles into specific points on the body to stimulate energy flow and promote healing. It has been shown to be effective for reducing pain, including neuropathic pain.
- **Neurologist:** A neurologist specializes in diagnosing and treating disorders of the nervous system, including neuropathy. They can assess the extent of nerve damage, determine the underlying cause, and recommend appropriate treatments.

- **Psychologist or Therapist:** Chronic pain can take a toll on emotional and mental well-being. A psychologist or therapist can provide support, teach coping mechanisms, and help you develop strategies for managing stress, anxiety, and depression.

By working collaboratively, we can create a comprehensive and personalized treatment plan that addresses the root causes of your neuropathy, manages your pain effectively, and empowers you to regain function and improve your overall quality of life.

Exploring Alternative Medications for Neuropathic Pain

While opioids were once the go-to solution for neuropathic pain, the growing awareness of their risks and limitations has led to a greater emphasis on safer, non-opioid medications that can provide effective pain relief without the risk of dependence and addiction.

Here are some commonly used non-opioid medications for neuropathic pain:

1. Topical Pain Relief: Soothing Nerves From the Outside In

Topical creams, gels, and patches can provide localized pain relief by directly targeting the affected nerves. They're often a good option for those seeking to minimize systemic side effects.

- **Capsaicin Cream:** Capsaicin, the compound that gives chili peppers their heat, works by depleting a neurotransmitter called substance P, which is involved in transmitting pain signals. While capsaicin cream can cause initial burning or stinging, with regular use, it can desensitize nerves and reduce pain.
- **Lidocaine Patches:** Lidocaine is a local anesthetic that blocks nerve signals, providing numbness and pain relief. Lidocaine patches are often used for localized neuropathic pain, such as that caused by shingles (post-herpetic neuralgia).

2. NMDA Receptor Antagonists: Interrupting Pain Signals

NMDA receptors are involved in transmitting pain signals in the spinal cord and brain. NMDA receptor antagonists work by blocking these receptors, reducing pain perception.

- **Memantine:** Originally developed for Alzheimer's disease, memantine has shown promise in treating neuropathic pain. It's believed to work by reducing the excitability of nerve cells involved in pain transmission.

3. Sodium Channel Blockers: Calming Overactive Nerves

Sodium channels are essential for nerve cell communication. When nerves are damaged, these channels can become overactive, leading to increased pain signaling. Sodium channel blockers work by stabilizing these channels, reducing nerve excitability and pain.

- **Carbamazepine:** While traditionally used as an anticonvulsant for epilepsy, carbamazepine can also be effective for certain types of neuropathic pain, particularly trigeminal neuralgia (a condition causing intense facial pain).
- **Mexiletine:** This medication, also used for heart rhythm disorders, can help reduce pain in some individuals with neuropathic pain.

Think of neuropathic pain medications as tools in a toolbox – each designed for a specific task.

Unfortunately, finding the right tool often involves trying several until you discover one that perfectly fits your individual needs. That's why it's vital to team up with your doctor. They'll help you select the right tools, track your progress, and make adjustments along the way, so you can find lasting relief.

Unlocking the Power of Non-Drug Therapies

While medications can play a role in managing neuropathy pain, a truly holistic approach often incorporates non-pharmacological therapies that address the multifaceted nature of this condition. These therapies, often used in conjunction with medications, can provide lasting relief, improve function, and enhance overall well-being without the risks of side effects or dependence associated with long-term medication use.

1. Chiropractic Care: Restoring Alignment and Nerve Flow

Chiropractic care focuses on the relationship between the spine and the nervous system, recognizing that misalignments in the spine can interfere with nerve function and contribute to pain and other symptoms.

- **Spinal Adjustments:** Chiropractors use gentle, hands-on techniques called adjustments to realign the vertebrae in the spine, restoring proper nerve flow and reducing nerve irritation.

- **Complementary Therapies:** Many chiropractors also incorporate other therapies, such as massage, stretching, and rehabilitative exercises, to address muscle imbalances, improve flexibility, and support overall musculoskeletal health.

2. Physical Therapy: Strengthening, Stretching, and Re-Educating

Physical therapy plays a crucial role in restoring strength, flexibility, balance, and coordination, helping individuals with neuropathy regain function and improve their quality of life.

- **Targeted Exercises:** Physical therapists design personalized exercise programs to strengthen weakened muscles, improve range of motion, and enhance balance and coordination.
- **TENS Therapy:** Transcutaneous electrical nerve stimulation (TENS) uses a small, battery-powered device to deliver electrical impulses to the affected nerves, blocking pain signals and providing relief.

3. Cognitive Behavioral Therapy (CBT): Retraining Your Brain

Imagine chronic pain as a shadow constantly looming over you. It can cloud your mood, trigger fear and worry, making you feel trapped. But with CBT, you learn how to break free from those shadows. You'll discover how to shift your mindset and adjust your habits to reduce pain perception and regain control of your life.

- **Pain Management Strategies:** CBT teaches you coping mechanisms, relaxation techniques, and strategies for managing pain flare-ups, empowering you to regain a sense of control over your experience.

4. Mindfulness and Meditation: Finding Calm Amidst the Storm

Mindfulness and meditation practices cultivate present-moment awareness, helping you detach from pain sensations, reduce stress, and enhance your overall sense of well-being.

- **Mindful Breathing:** Simple deep breathing exercises can calm the nervous system, reduce muscle tension, and shift your focus away from pain.

- **Guided Meditation:** Guided meditations specifically designed for pain management can help you visualize healing, reduce stress, and cultivate a sense of peace.

5. Acupuncture: Restoring Energy Flow

Acupuncture, a traditional Chinese medicine practice, involves inserting thin needles into specific points on the body to stimulate energy flow (Qi) and promote healing.

- **Pain Relief:** Acupuncture has been shown to be effective for reducing pain, including neuropathic pain, by modulating pain signals in the brain and spinal cord.

6. Yoga and Tai Chi: Gentle Movement for Body and Mind

Yoga and tai chi are gentle mind-body practices that combine physical postures, controlled breathing, and mindfulness to enhance flexibility, improve balance, reduce stress, and promote relaxation.

- **Adaptable Practices:** Many yoga and tai chi poses can be modified to accommodate physical limitations, making them accessible for individuals with neuropathy.

Neuropathy doesn't just impact your body; it can throw your emotional world into turmoil too. These non-pharmaceutical therapies provide a lifeline, offering holistic support to manage the physical, emotional, and psychological impact of this condition. By working with your body's innate healing capabilities, you can regain a sense of control, cultivate inner peace, and experience a renewed sense of energy and well-being.

The WARRIOR Protocol: Your Personalized Path to Neuropathy Relief

Neuropathy treatment doesn't have to be solely about managing symptoms with pills. WARRIOR offers a holistic, non-invasive approach that seeks to tackle the root causes of the condition. It's a personalized plan combining innovative therapies with ancient healing wisdom to empower your body's own natural healing potential.

Here's how the WARRIOR Protocol can be an effective part of your neuropathy pain management plan:

1. Hako-Med Electromedicine: Awakening Nerve Regeneration

Hako-Med Electromedicine, also known as Horizontal Therapy, utilizes gentle electrical impulses to stimulate nerve regeneration, improve circulation, and reduce pain. It's like a gentle nudge to your nervous system, encouraging it to repair and restore optimal function.

- **Enhanced Blood Flow:** Hako-Med therapy promotes vasodilation—the widening of blood vessels—improving blood flow to the affected nerves, delivering vital oxygen and nutrients essential for healing.
- **Accelerated Tissue Regeneration:** The gentle electrical stimulation encourages cell regeneration and repair, helping to rebuild damaged nerve tissues.
- **Reduced Pain and Inflammation:** Hako-Med therapy can help modulate pain signals and reduce inflammation, providing much-needed relief while addressing the underlying causes of neuropathy.

2. Infrared Light Therapy: Harnessing the Healing Power of Light

Infrared Light Therapy uses specific wavelengths of light to penetrate deep into tissues, promoting healing and reducing inflammation. It's like bathing your nerves in a soothing, restorative light.

- **Stimulated Cellular Repair:** Infrared light stimulates cellular activity, enhancing the production of ATP (adenosine triphosphate), the energy currency of your cells. This boost in energy production supports nerve cell regeneration and repair.
- **Reduced Inflammation:** Infrared light has anti-inflammatory properties, helping to calm inflammation in and around the nerves, reducing pain and promoting healing.

3. Vibration Therapy: Shaking Things Up for Better Circulation

Vibration therapy uses gentle vibrations to stimulate blood flow, relax muscles, and improve nerve function. It's like a gentle massage for your nerves, encouraging circulation and promoting relaxation.

- **Enhanced Blood Flow:** The vibrations help improve circulation, delivering oxygen and nutrients to the nerves and removing waste products.
- **Reduced Muscle Tension:** Vibration therapy can help relax tight muscles, which can often compress or irritate nerves, contributing to pain and dysfunction.

4. Electrostimulation: Re-educating Muscles and Nerves

Targeted electrostimulation therapies can be used to re-educate muscles, improve coordination, and reduce pain.

- **Muscle Re-Education:** Electrostimulation can help activate weakened muscles, improving strength and coordination.
- **Pain Modulation:** The electrical impulses can help block pain signals, providing relief and interrupting pain cycles.

5. SoftWave Therapy: Awakening Your Body's Healing Potential

SoftWave Therapy is a revolutionary, non-invasive technology that harnesses the power of acoustic waves to stimulate healing, reduce inflammation, and restore optimal function. It's a gentle yet powerful approach that can significantly enhance the lives of those struggling with neuropathy.

- **Supercharged Circulation:** SoftWave therapy dramatically increases blood supply to the treated area—by up to 300%—delivering a surge of oxygen and nutrients to nourish damaged nerves and accelerate healing.
- **Inflammation Control:** The acoustic waves effectively modulate inflammation, calming the internal fire that contributes to nerve damage and pain.
- **Stem Cell Activation:** SoftWave therapy has a unique ability to stimulate and activate stem cells, your body's own repair and regeneration specialists. These activated stem cells migrate to the site of injury, promoting tissue repair and restoring function.
- **Tissue Regeneration:** The gentle acoustic waves promote tissue regeneration, helping to rebuild damaged nerves and restore their structural integrity.
- **Pain Relief:** SoftWave therapy is effective for reducing both acute and chronic pain,

providing much-needed relief while addressing the underlying causes of neuropathy.

The WARRIOR Protocol integrates these non-invasive therapies to create a comprehensive and personalized approach to neuropathy care. By addressing the root causes, promoting nerve regeneration, and reducing pain, it empowers your body to heal naturally and reclaim a life of greater comfort, mobility, and vitality.

Breaking Free from Opioids: A Safe and Supported Approach

If you've been taking opioids for an extended period, especially for chronic pain like neuropathy, you might be physically dependent on the medication. This means your body has adapted to the presence of the drug, and abruptly stopping it can lead to withdrawal symptoms, which can range from uncomfortable to severe.

Never Stop Opioids Cold Turkey:

It's crucial to understand that abruptly stopping opioids without medical supervision is dangerous and can lead to severe withdrawal symptoms, including:

- **Intense Pain:** Your original pain might return with a vengeance, often feeling even worse than before you started taking opioids.
- **Flu-like Symptoms:** You might experience nausea, vomiting, diarrhea, muscle aches, chills, sweating, and a runny nose.
- **Anxiety and Insomnia:** Opioid withdrawal often triggers anxiety, restlessness, and difficulty sleeping.
- **Dangerous Complications:** In severe cases, withdrawal can lead to seizures, dehydration, or heart problems.

Tapering: A Gradual Path to Freedom

The safest and most effective way to discontinue opioids is through a gradual tapering process, conducted under the guidance of your healthcare provider.

- **Personalized Tapering Schedule:** Your doctor will work with you to create a personalized tapering schedule, slowly reducing your opioid dosage over time. This allows your body to adjust gradually and minimizes withdrawal symptoms.
- **Supportive Medications:** Your doctor might prescribe medications to help manage

withdrawal symptoms, such as anti-nausea medications, muscle relaxants, or medications to aid sleep.
- **Non-Drug Therapies:** Incorporating non-drug therapies, like acupuncture, massage, or physical therapy, can help reduce pain, ease withdrawal symptoms, and promote relaxation.

Seeking Help for Opioid Addiction:

If you're struggling with opioid addiction, it's essential to seek professional help. Addiction is a treatable brain disease, and recovery is possible with the right support.

- **Addiction Treatment Centers:** Addiction treatment centers offer a range of programs, including detoxification, inpatient and outpatient treatment, counseling, and support groups.
- **Support Groups:** Support groups, such as Narcotics Anonymous (NA), provide a safe and supportive space for individuals recovering from opioid addiction.
- **National Helpline:** The Substance Abuse and Mental Health Services Administration (SAMHSA) National Helpline provides free,

confidential, 24/7 support for individuals and families facing mental health and substance use disorders. You can reach them at 1-800-662-HELP (4357).

Kicking an opioid dependence or addiction isn't easy. It takes a ton of strength, support, and a deep desire to heal. But you don't have to go through it alone. Your healthcare provider is there for you. There are amazing support groups where people understand exactly what you're going through. And national helplines are always just a phone call away. There is light at the end of the tunnel, and help is within reach.

Your Voice Matters: Talking to Your Doctor About Pain Management

When it comes to your health, you are your own best advocate. This is especially true when discussing pain management options with your healthcare provider. Open, honest, and informed communication is crucial for ensuring you receive the most appropriate and effective care for your neuropathy.

Embrace Open Dialogue:

Don't be afraid to share your concerns, ask questions, and advocate for your needs. Your doctor is there to help you, but they can only provide the best care if they understand your experiences, preferences, and goals.

Questions to Guide the Conversation:

Here are some key questions to ask your doctor about pain management options, particularly regarding opioids and alternatives:

- **What are the potential benefits and risks of opioids for my type of neuropathy?**
- **Are there non-opioid medications that might be effective for my pain?**
- **What non-drug therapies might be helpful for managing my pain and improving my function?**
- **What are the potential side effects of the medications or therapies you're recommending?**
- **How will we monitor my progress and adjust my treatment plan if needed?**
- **What are the risks of long-term opioid use, and how can we minimize those risks?**
- **If I'm concerned about opioid dependence or addiction, what resources are available to support me?**

Your Right to a Second Opinion:

Remember, you always have the right to seek a second opinion if you're unsure about your diagnosis, your treatment options, or if you feel your concerns aren't being addressed. Getting another perspective can provide you with valuable information, reassurance, and alternative approaches to consider.

The Power of Empowerment:

Taking an active role in your healthcare journey empowers you to make informed decisions, advocate for your needs, and partner with your healthcare providers to create a treatment plan that aligns with your values and health goals. Remember, your voice matters, and your well-being is worth advocating for.

The opioid epidemic has exposed the limitations of relying solely on medications for pain relief. It has also sparked innovation and a renewed focus on developing safer, more effective, and sustainable solutions for chronic pain. By embracing a holistic approach, prioritizing research, and fostering open communication between patients and healthcare providers, we can create a brighter future for those living with neuropathy and chronic pain.

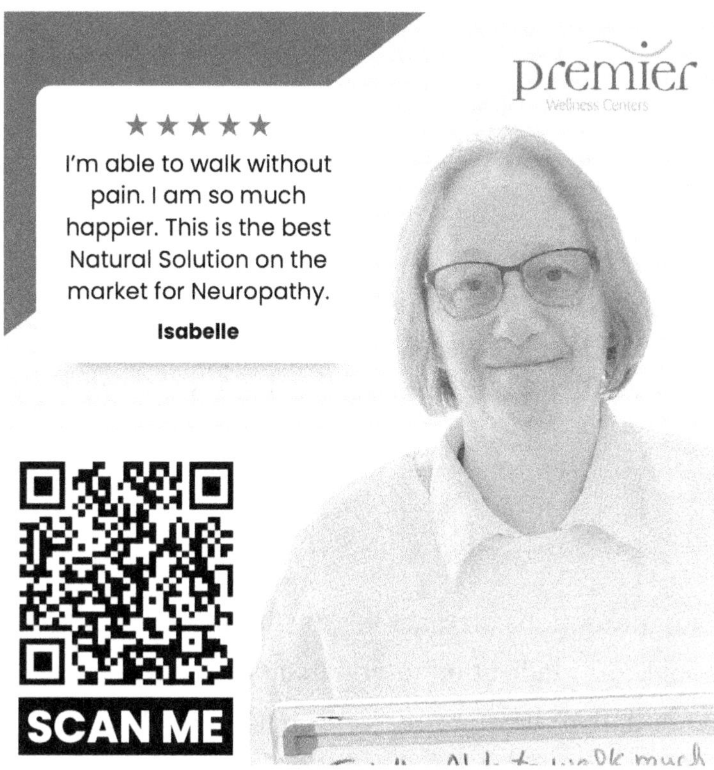

** Every patient's journey is unique. This testimonial does not guarantee similar results for others.*

Unlock Your Path to Neuropathy Relief Now: Dial (772) 279-4145 to Speak With a Skilled Neuropathy Professional Today!

Individual results may vary. Please review the disclaimer after the Table of Contents.

12

YOUR JOURNEY TO RELIEF STARTS NOW: TAKING THE FIRST STEPS WITH THE WARRIOR PROTOCOL

Congratulations on reaching the final chapter of this book! Your dedication to understanding and potentially relieving your neuropathy is truly inspiring. You've gained valuable insights into the complexities of this condition, the limitations of conventional treatments, and the potential for lasting relief through the holistic approach of the WARRIOR method.

Now, are you ready to turn that knowledge into action and experience the transformative power of WARRIOR firsthand? Click here to schedule a consultation today, or call us at (772) 279-4145.

A few years ago, a gentleman named Robert came to PWC feeling hopeless. Years of battling neuropathy had taken their toll, and he was struggling to find lasting relief. However, after embracing the WARRIOR Protocol, he experienced a remarkable transformation. The burning pain subsided, the numbness receded, and he was able to reclaim a life of greater comfort, mobility, and joy.

While it's important to remember that individual results may vary, Robert's story is a testament to the power of this holistic approach to healing neuropathy.

I'm also excited to invite you to my "**3 Secrets to Relieving Neuropathy Naturally**" masterclass—a comprehensive online program designed to equip you with the knowledge, strategies, and support you need to regain control of your health and reclaim a life of vitality and well-being.

In This Transformative Masterclass, You'll Discover:

- The 3 Breakthrough Secrets to Healing Neuropathy:
    1. **Oxygen & Angiogenesis:** We'll delve into the crucial role of blood flow and oxygen supply for nerve health. You'll learn how to improve circulation and stimulate the growth of new blood vessels (angiogenesis) through dietary changes,

targeted supplements, and lifestyle modifications.

2. **Inflammatory Regulation:** We'll explore the damaging effects of chronic inflammation on your nerves and empower you with strategies to calm the fire within, including an anti-inflammatory diet, stress management techniques, and natural supplements.

3. **Ignite Nerve Healing:** We'll unlock the secrets to providing your body with the resources it needs to repair and regenerate nerves, including specific nutrients, targeted therapies, and gentle exercises to stimulate nerve function.

- The 3 R's of Lasting Relief:
  1. **REMOVE:** Identify and eliminate the factors contributing to your neuropathy, whether it's inflammatory foods, chronic stress, underlying health conditions, or unhealthy habits.

  2. **RESTORE:** Nourish your body with the building blocks it needs to heal and regenerate, embracing an anti-inflammatory diet, targeted supplements, and therapies that promote nerve regeneration.

3. **RETAIN:** Create lasting lifestyle changes to maintain nerve health, prevent future damage, and support your overall well-being.

By joining the masterclass, you'll gain a deeper understanding of neuropathy and the often-hidden factors that contribute to its development. You'll go beyond simply managing symptoms and learn practical, evidence-based strategies to reduce pain, improve nerve function, and enhance your overall quality of life.

We'll explore a holistic approach that addresses not just the physical aspects of neuropathy but also the emotional and lifestyle factors that play a crucial role in your healing journey. Plus, you'll connect with a supportive community of individuals who understand your challenges and can offer encouragement and inspiration along the way. Most importantly, you'll reignite your hope and empower yourself to take control of your health, creating a brighter, healthier future.

Scan the code below to join the masterclass and begin your transformative journey toward lasting relief!

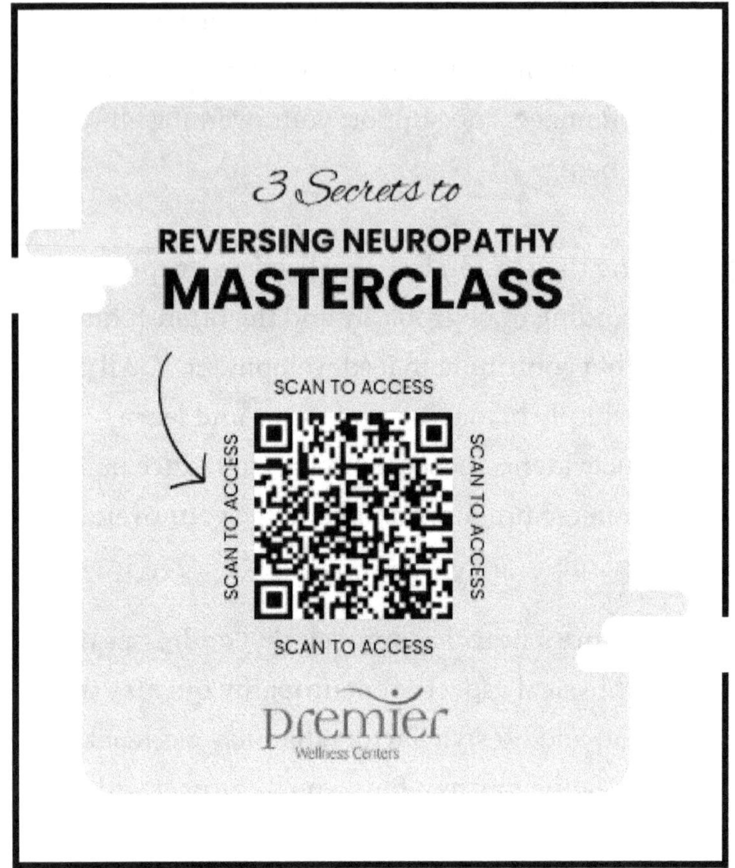

Ready for Personalized Support?

Our dedicated team provides comprehensive and personalized care to help you achieve greater well-being and reclaim your vitality. Scan the code below to schedule a consultation and discover how we can tailor a personalized treatment plan to meet your unique needs. Please note that scheduling a consultation does not guarantee specific results, as each individual's condition and response to treatment vary.

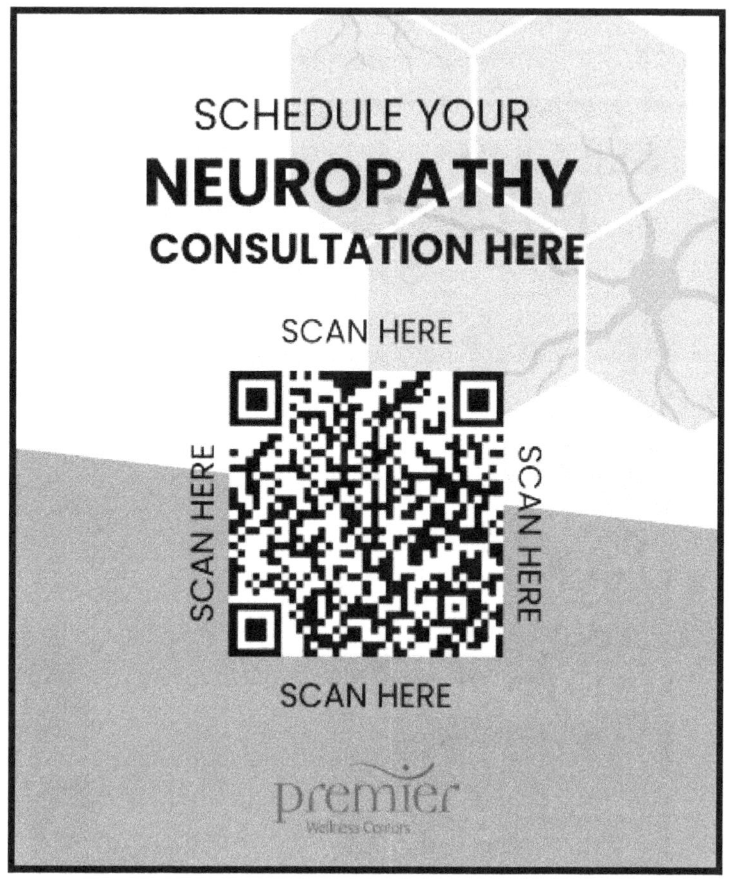

My hope is that this book has ignited a spark of possibility within you—a realization that you don't have to simply "live with" neuropathy. The power to heal lies within your own body, and the WARRIOR

Protocol, combined with the knowledge you've gained from this book, can guide you on that journey. We look forward to welcoming you to the Premier Wellness Centers community and supporting you every step of the way.

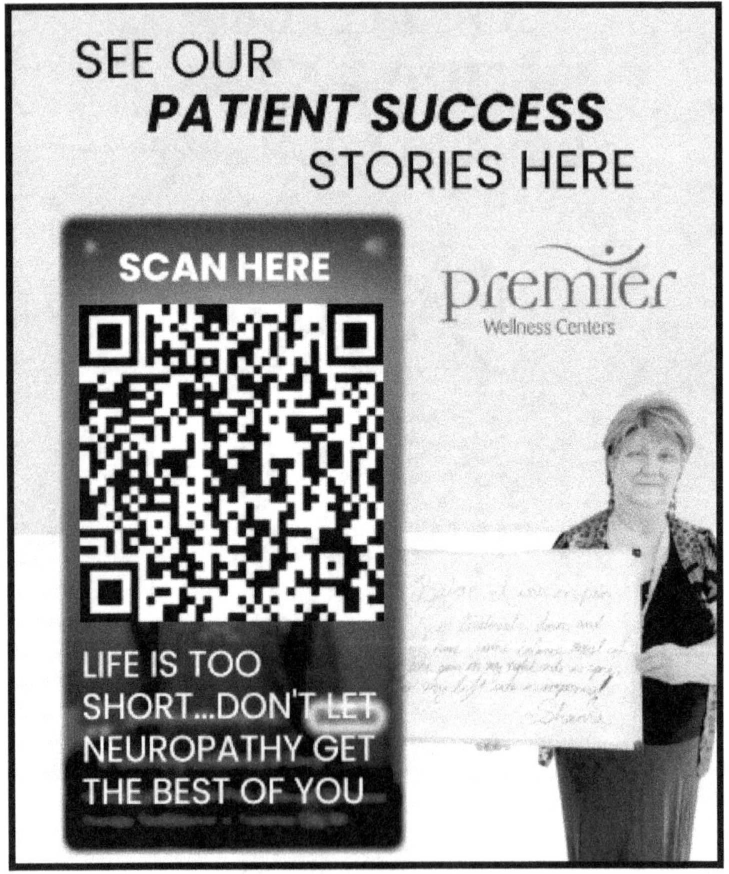

Individual results may vary.

Congratulations on completing this transformative journey through these pages! By taking this step, you've not only educated yourself but also taken a proactive stand for your health, your happiness, and your future. I hope you've embraced the free tools, resources, and assets in each chapter and found them to be valuable allies in your healing journey.

Remember, you are not alone in this process. You are part of a growing community of WARRIORS reclaiming their lives and rewriting their stories beyond neuropathy. My deepest wish for you is a future filled with strength, vitality, and joy—a life where hope replaces despair and freedom replaces limitations.

You've already taken the most important step: believing in the possibility of change. As you continue forward, may you find blessings, breakthroughs, and the health you deserve. Here's to your brighter, healthier tomorrow! Welcome to the Premier Wellness Centers family—we are here to support you every step of the way. Now, go forward with confidence and courage. The best is yet to come! Dr. Bill Jensen DC.